T0075444

Funding Global Health Engagement to Support the Geographic Combatant Commands

BETH GRILL, TRUPTI BRAHMBHATT, PAULINE MOORE,
JENNIFER D. P. MORONEY, CHANDLER SACHS

Prepared for the Office of the Assistant Secretary of Defense for Health Affairs
Approved for public release; distribution unlimited

 NATIONAL DEFENSE RESEARCH INSTITUTE

For more information on this publication, visit **www.rand.org/t/RRA1357-2**.

About RAND

The RAND Corporation is a research organization that develops solutions to public policy challenges to help make communities throughout the world safer and more secure, healthier and more prosperous. RAND is nonprofit, nonpartisan, and committed to the public interest. To learn more about RAND, visit www.rand.org.

Research Integrity

Our mission to help improve policy and decisionmaking through research and analysis is enabled through our core values of quality and objectivity and our unwavering commitment to the highest level of integrity and ethical behavior. To help ensure our research and analysis are rigorous, objective, and nonpartisan, we subject our research publications to a robust and exacting quality-assurance process; avoid both the appearance and reality of financial and other conflicts of interest through staff training, project screening, and a policy of mandatory disclosure; and pursue transparency in our research engagements through our commitment to the open publication of our research findings and recommendations, disclosure of the source of funding of published research, and policies to ensure intellectual independence. For more information, visit www.rand.org/about/research-integrity.

RAND's publications do not necessarily reflect the opinions of its research clients and sponsors.

Published by the RAND Corporation, Santa Monica, Calif.
© 2023 RAND Corporation
RAND® is a registered trademark.

Library of Congress Cataloging-in-Publication Data is available for this publication.

ISBN: 978-1-9774-1005-4

Cover: U.S. Army Photo by Sgt. 1st Class Elena Chung.

Limited Print and Electronic Distribution Rights

About This Report

The combined challenges that the U.S. Department of Defense (DoD) faces in addressing the coronavirus disease 2019 (COVID-19) pandemic and preparing for a potential conflict with a near-peer adversary have made the need to protect the health and safety of U.S. forces more acute. Global health engagement (GHE) provides an important mechanism to work with allies and partners to develop their medical capacity and medical support capabilities and improve U.S. interoperability with them to help ensure U.S. force protection and medical readiness. Although the defense community has a broad remit to engage in global health activities with partner nations for the purpose of improving the health and safety of U.S. warfighters, it has not integrated GHE into combatant command operational or security cooperation planning, nor has it provided consistent funding for these activities.

A 2018 GHE capabilities-based assessment (CBA), funded by the Deputy Assistant Secretary of Defense for Health Readiness Policy and Oversight, identified shortfalls related to an inadequate awareness and understanding of GHE as a tool for achieving combatant command objectives. The study found substantial gaps in the way DoD, organizes, manages, resources, and develops its workforce for GHE and highlighted DoD's lack of funding to support and sustain GHE priority activities in support of long-term objectives. To close the CBA-identified gaps, a DOTmLPF-P[1] Change Recommendation was generated with recommendations that were endorsed via a Joint Requirements Oversight Committee Memorandum, and the overall responsibility for actions was assigned to the Office of the Deputy Assistant Secretary of Defense (DASD) for Health Readiness Policy and Oversight. OASD Health Affairs asked RAND researchers to conduct research and analysis in support of actions related to education and training, the feasibility of an Intellipedia-like site, technology platforms, and dedicated funding mechanisms.

This report presents research conducted in support of the funding task. To address this task, we identified the evolving GHE priorities of five of the six geographic combatant commands (GCCs), as well as their activities, sources of funding, and the challenges they face in supporting their objectives. We reviewed the relevant GHE instructions and policies and engaged in discussion with more than 75 DoD policy and service leaders and members of the medical community in five GCCs and their service components, as well as members of the policy, legal, and financial communities across DoD. Using these discussions and a series of follow-up group discussions, we proposed several courses of action for providing more-targeted resources to conduct GHE activities in support of GCC objectives. This report should be of interest to the

---

[1] DOTmLPF-P stands for Doctrine, Organization, Training, materiel, Leadership and education, Personnel, Facilities, and Policy.

Joint Staff and strategic planners in the GHE community, as well as officials in the larger DoD medical and security cooperation communities.

This report is part of a series of three reports. The two companion reports detail the findings of our other study tasks, which address the feasibility of an Intellipedia-like platform for GHE and the education and training of the DoD workforce for global health engagements.

The research reported here was completed in August 2022 and underwent security review with the sponsor and the Defense Office of Prepublication and Security Review before public release.

RAND National Security Research Division

This research was sponsored by the Office of the Assistant Secretary of Defense for Health Affairs and conducted within the Personnel, Readiness, and Health Program of the RAND National Security Research Division (NSRD), which operates the National Defense Research Institute (NDRI), a federally funded research and development center sponsored by the Office of the Secretary of Defense, the Joint Staff, the Unified Combatant Commands, the Navy, the Marine Corps, the defense agencies, and the defense intelligence enterprise.

For more information on the RAND Personnel, Readiness, and Health Program, see www.rand.org/nsrd/prh or contact the director (contact information is provided on the webpage).

Acknowledgments

We would like to offer special thanks to our project monitor at DASD Health Readiness Policy and Oversight, Dr. J. Christopher Daniel, for his guidance and support throughout the course of this study. Dr. Daniel's extensive knowledge and experience and keen interest in GHE was critical to our study. We would also like to thank the leaders and staffs of the Joint Staff Surgeon for sharing their time and insight with us. This project benefited a great deal from conversations with individuals from across the GHE community, services, GCCs, and DoD education and training programs, as well as DoD financial, legal, and congressional affairs offices. We are indebted to the combatant command and service component command surgeons and their staffs, who generously shared their time and expertise with us throughout our study. Although we cannot mention them by name, their contributions were invaluable to our analysis. We are also grateful for our reviewers, Wesley Palmer, Brent Thomas, and Sarah Meadows, for their helpful suggestions that greatly improved the quality of our written work. Finally, we would like to thank Maria Falvo for her assistance in preparing this report and our editor, Brian Dau.

Summary

Global health engagement (GHE) provides a mechanism for the U.S. Department of Defense (DoD) to work with U.S. allies and partners to develop their medical capacity and medical support capabilities and to improve U.S. interoperability with them, which can be critical to ensuring the health and safety of U.S. warfighters. Military medical personnel have a broad remit to engage individually or as a unit with a partner's armed forces or civilian authorities to increase partner-nation health capabilities and capacity. The purpose of these engagements includes maintaining both U.S. force protection and medical readiness to respond to contingencies and the ability of U.S. forces to achieve a variety of U.S. national security objectives.[2]

Although the scope of global health activities has expanded significantly since the end of the Cold War, there are no dedicated sources of GHE funding. Currently, GHE activities are funded through a variety of funding mechanisms that were designed for a variety of purposes. Moreover, many GHE stakeholders have difficulty demonstrating to strategic planners at the geographic combatant commands (GCCs) how GHE directly supports combatant command plans and other strategic plans. Medical planners often rely on various one-time or single-year security cooperation funds, which makes it difficult to support sustained and consistent engagement. As DoD confronts evolving challenges posed by the coronavirus disease 2019 (COVID-19) pandemic and the threat of conflict with a near-peer competitor, the need to prioritize resources for GHE to ensure U.S. medical readiness and force protection has become more acute.[3]

The Deputy Assistant Secretary of Defense (DASD) for Health Readiness Policy and Oversight addressed some of these challenges in a 2018 GHE capabilities-based assessment (CBA) aimed at facilitating the efficient conduct of GHE activities to meet combatant command

---

[2] GHE activities have expanded to include support for U.S. stability operations in Afghanistan and Iraq, humanitarian assistance in response to disasters in South America and the Pacific, preventive medicine campaigns in Africa, and biological threat reduction efforts in Eastern Europe and throughout the world. DoD Instruction 2000.30 stipulates that GHE is a tool to achieve a variety of national security objectives. It also notes that GHE activities should be prioritized to "(a) build the capacity of the PN [partner-nation] government to maintain a level of health care conducive to a healthy population, (b) bolster the civilian population's confidence in PN governance, and (c) lower the PN's susceptibility to destabilizing influences" (Department of Defense Instruction 2000.30, *Global Health Engagement (GHE) Activities*, U.S. Department of Defense, July 12, 2017, p. 5).

[3] For information on the future demands for casualty care in a potential conflict with near-peer adversaries and the relevance of GHE in preparing for these operations, see Brent Thomas, *Preparing for the Future of Combat Casualty Care: Opportunities to Refine the Military Health System's Alignment with the National Defense Strategy*, RAND Corporation, RR-A713-1, 2021.

objectives.[4] To close the CBA-identified gaps, a DOTmLPF-P[5] Change Recommendation was generated listing recommendations across the DOTmLPF-P spectrum, which were endorsed via a Joint Requirements Oversight Committee Memorandum. Overall responsibility for implementing these recommendations was assigned to the Office of the Deputy Assistant Secretary of Defense (DASD) for Health Readiness Policy and Oversight.[6] OASD Health Affairs asked RAND researchers to conduct research and analysis in support of the following actions related to gaps in the preparation of and support for U.S. forces conducting GHE and the tracking of GHE activities: (1) synchronizing GHE training and education, (2) orchestrating funding mechanisms to enable long-term global health capability, and (3) using the most-efficient technology platforms. This report presents the results of our research related to GHE funding mechanisms.[7]

Research Approach

We adopted a strategic approach to analyzing GHE funding mechanisms and their ability to enable long-term GHE capability development. Given the CBA's focus on meeting combatant command objectives, we looked primarily at GHE funding mechanisms that were under GCC influence or control. We began by first identifying GHE priorities for meeting combatant command objectives, current GHE activities, and existing funding mechanisms. We then focused on documenting the challenges that GHE stakeholders face in meeting GCC objectives. We conducted a series of discussions with more than 75 officials in the command surgeons' offices across five of the six GCCs and U.S. Air Force components, then conducted a deep-dive analysis on the U.S. Indo-Pacific Command (INDOPACOM) region, interviewing personnel and analyzing data from each of the component commands.[8] Because of a lack of comprehensive data available on DoD's engagement in global health, we drew heavily on these discussions for the analysis. We validated our findings by conducting two virtual group discussion events that

---

[4] DoD, *Global Health Engagement (GHE) Capabilities-Based Assessment (CBA) Study*, July 23, 2018, Not available to the general public.

[5] DOTmLPF-P stands for Doctrine, Organization, Training, materiel, Leadership and education, Personnel, Facilities, and Policy.

[6] Paul Selva, Vice Chairman of the Joint Chiefs of Staff, "DOTmLPF-P Change Recommendation for Global Health Engagement," memorandum, JROCM 008-19, February 25, 2019, Not available to the general public.

[7] The two other reports in this series are Jefferson P. Marquis, Trupti Brahmbhatt, Aaron Clark-Ginsberg, Victoria M. Smith, and David E. Thaler, *Educating and Training the Department of Defense Workforce for Global Health Engagement to Support the Geographic Combatant Commands*, RAND Corporation, RR-A1357-1, 2023; and Padmaja Vedula, Trupti Brahmbhatt, Jonathan Tran, and Chandler Sachs, *Assessing Technology Platforms for Global Health Engagement to Support Integration of Efforts Across Geographic Combatant Commands*, RAND Corporation, RR-A1357-3, 2023.

[8] Because of time constraints, we were only able to interview representatives from one service component across all commands. We selected the Air Force because of our contacts within the Department of the Air Force. However, we were able to capture the insights of each of the service components in the INDOPACOM area of responsibility, where we conducted a more in-depth analysis. We selected INDOPACOM for a deep dive because of the region's growing strategic importance in U.S. defense policy.

brought together military medical personnel from across the GCCs, as well as members of the policy, legal, and financial communities across DoD. We then held follow-up discussions with DoD officials in the Office of the Secretary of Defense, the Joint Staff, and a combatant command planner in the Strategy, Policy, and Plans Directorate (J5).

This study was conducted from 2020 to 2021, when travel restrictions related to the COVID-19 pandemic precluded us from conducting in-person discussions. All individual and group discussions were therefore conducted virtually. The pandemic was a limiting factor in our analysis, because some DoD personnel had limited experience or data from the pre-pandemic era. Yet the pandemic also proved to be a benefit because it highlighted the importance of GHE in addressing public health concerns, as a means of both ensuring U.S. force protection and enhancing medical readiness and relationships with partner nations to meet theater objectives related to great-power competition.

Key Findings

Our analysis of DoD GHE priorities and funding mechanisms led to the following key findings:

- GHE priorities vary across the GCCs, as outlined in Table S.1.
- In the U.S European Command (EUCOM) and U.S. Central Command (CENTCOM), GHE efforts focus on expanding regional expeditionary medical capacity and trauma care support for current and potential operations.
- In the U.S. Southern Command (SOUTHCOM) and U.S. Africa Command (AFRICOM), GHE efforts relate to increasing partner capacity to respond to infectious diseases and public health needs and developing medical support capabilities for humanitarian assistance and peacekeeping missions.
- In INDOPACOM (for which we conducted a deep-dive analysis), GHE activities are focused both on enhancing public health and support for humanitarian disasters and increasingly on developing regional military medical capabilities in support of potential contingency operations.

Table S.1. GHE Priorities, Activities, and Sources of Funding Across the GCCs

GCC	GHE Priorities	Primary Activities	Primary Funding Sources
INDOPACOM	• Enhancing public health and support for humanitarian disasters • Providing access for potential contingencies • Increasing regional military medical capabilities	• Public health outreach • Disease surveillance and trauma care exchanges • Medical evacuation (MEDEVAC) and casualty evacuation (CASEVAC) exercises	• Asia Pacific Regional Initiative (APRI) • Overseas Humanitarian, Disaster, and Civic Aid (OHDACA) • Service Operation and Maintenance (O&M) funding
EUCOM	• Expanding expeditionary medical capacity • Increasing North Atlantic Treaty Organization (NATO) interoperability	• Role 1 and Role 2 capability expert exchanges[a] • Medical logistics exercises	• European Deterrence Initiative (EDI) • Traditional Combatant Command Activities (TCA)
CENTCOM	• Improving regional trauma care for current operations	• Trauma care facility support • Personnel exchanges and embeds • MEDEVAC exercises	• Foreign Military Sales (FMS) • TCA
AFRICOM	• Increasing partner capacity to respond to infectious diseases • Developing medical support capabilities for counterterrorism and peacekeeping	• Preventive medicine education and training • Partner CASEVAC and trauma care training	• President's Emergency Plan for AIDS Relief (PEPFAR) • Partnership for Regional East Africa Counterterrorism (PREACT) • Trans-Sahara Counterterrorism Partnership (TSCTP) • African Peacekeeping Rapid Response Partnership (APRRP)
SOUTHCOM	• Building regional medical response capabilities • Increasing public health capacity and opportunities for U.S. medical training	• Public health outreach • Medical Readiness Training Exercises (MEDRETEs)	• OHDACA • O&M funding

SOURCES: Features information from stakeholder discussions and GCC briefings.
[a] Role 1 capability is known as *first responder care* (providing immediate life-saving measures). Role 2 capability includes more-advanced trauma management and emergency medical treatment and provides a greater capability to resuscitate patients. Full definitions for Role 1 and Role 2 capabilities can be found in Joint Publication 4-02, *Joint Health Services*, Joint Chiefs of Staff, Incorporating Change 1, September 28, 2018.

- Despite differences in regional priorities, GCCs are increasingly focused on achieving U.S. force protection and medical readiness objectives.
  - The GCCs pursue different GHE activities according to their theater requirements, yet GCC representatives expressed a common interest in building partner capacity and developing interoperable medical capabilities to meet U.S. strategic objectives related to force protection and medical readiness.

- GHE funding is not prioritized to build partner-nation medical capacity or develop the interoperable medical capabilities necessary to meet future combatant command requirements for medical support.
    - GHE activities are supported by a variety of funding sources, which vary by region and purpose. There are no funding sources designed to support long-term GHE efforts for the purposes of meeting U.S. force protection or medical readiness objectives. Although there are some funding sources, such as OHDACA, that can be used over two years, there are no sources designated specifically for GHE. GHE activities are often conducted in concert with other security cooperation activities but are not prioritized for support. (Appendix A provides a list of current funding sources.)
    - A lack of reliable funding support has created significant barriers for GHE stakeholders. Medical planners across the GCCs noted that they are unable to build partner-nation medical capacity or develop the interoperable medical capabilities necessary to meet future combatant command requirements for medical support.
    - The operational requirements for medical support and demand for GHE are not yet incorporated into theater or service planning, making it difficult to prioritize funding for activities that support U.S. force protection and medical readiness.
    - Neither DoD nor Congress currently supports the establishment of a designated GHE funding source similar to a program of record in the DoD acquisition process.

Recommendations

Given these findings, we recommend that GHE focus on enhancing U.S. force health protection and medical readiness as a means of achieving GCC objectives. Specifically, we recommend that GHE become more closely integrated into GCC operational planning by identifying the demand for medical support and focusing GHE activities on building partner-nation capacity and capabilities to meet these demands. The first steps in this process are as follows:

- The GCC strategic planners (J5s) and command surgeons[9] should clarify the medical readiness and force protection requirements for their operational plans and identify how GHE can help meet these requirements.
- The GCCs, in coordination with the Joint Staff and Deputy Assistant Secretary of Defense (DASD) for Global Partnerships (GP) should develop regionally specific GHE plans based on operational requirements.

At the same time, it will be important to evaluate how well GCC objectives are being met under current security cooperation funding sources. Although there is consensus among GHE stakeholders on the need for dedicated multiyear funding to develop partner-nation medical

---

[9] Some GCCs and service components at GCCs use the term *surgeon general*, as opposed to *command surgeon*.

capacity and interoperable medical capabilities, it will be important to determine the extent to which GHE contributes to the achievement of GCC operational objectives and the extent to which these objectives are able to support (or fail to support) U.S. strategic goals.

DASD/GP should consider ways to incorporate GHE into its security cooperation evaluation and learning agenda.[10] This would draw greater attention and resources for the assessment, monitoring, and evaluation of medical- and health-related security cooperation activities on a regional and country basis. Such a move would help inform future GHE funding decisions and strengthen linkages with the J5 community writ large. Specifically, evaluation results will help inform the support base for future GHE, strengthen the links with GCC plans, and make it easier for GHE to compete for funding.

Until GHE is better understood as meeting an operational imperative and directly supporting GCC objectives, it will be difficult to establish a case for creating a new, dedicated source of funding for GHE. Thus, we recommend that DASD/GP **continue to leverage existing security cooperation mechanisms to support GHE, even while it pursues dedicated GHE funding to increase partner-nation capacity and capabilities to ensure the health and safety of U.S. forces.** We also identify additional options for DoD to use **existing funding mechanisms** to effectively meet current and future combatant command GHE requirements. These options include the following:

- Regional funding sources, such as the EDI or Pacific Deterrence Initiative (PDI) could be used to support partner-nation capacity-building and medical support infrastructure if GHE is designated as an operational requirement to support U.S. posture.
- Partnership capacity-building funds, such as the Section 333 program, could be used for GHE if health support is recognized as a component of an existing mission or institutional capacity-building.
- An expansion of Defense Health Program funding to support GHE activities aimed at developing partner-nation medical capacity for the purpose of protecting the health of U.S. forces.
- Designated support for GHE could be provided through service O&M funding for medical readiness. Such funding could support combined training and exercises with allies and partners to support U.S. medical readiness and resiliency.

Each of these funding options could help to address the need for more-consistent support to meet GCC priorities for medical support. However, each offers different benefits and limitations in terms of flexibility and scope, as well as the availability and likelihood of support. None of the options are mutually exclusive; in fact, it will be necessary to pursue multiple sources of funding to ensure that diverse needs for force protection and medical readiness are addressed. The most

---

[10] In fiscal year 2022, DoD "is transitioning from an annual strategic evaluation plan to a comprehensive learning agenda framework," which "identifies the most urgent knowledge gaps in the security cooperation (SC) community and then plans and prioritizes evidence-building activities to help fill these gaps" (DoD, "2022 Learning and Evaluation Agenda for Partnerships Framework," August 25, 2022, p. 1). The program, which was established by DASD/GP, is being conducted in coordination with the Defense Security Cooperation University.

effective way to designate funding for GHE and to prioritize engagement with allies and partners will depend on combatant command objectives and priorities and the likelihood of support from across the DoD community and Congress.

Contents

Figure and Tables

Figure

Tables

Chapter 1. Introduction

U.S. Department of Defense (DoD) global health engagement (GHE) is defined broadly as any health-related

> [i]nteraction between individuals or elements of DoD and those of a PN's [partner nation's] armed forces or civilian authorities, in coordination with other U.S. Government departments and agencies, to build trust and confidence, share information, coordinate mutual activities, maintain influence, and achieve interoperability in health-related activities that support U.S. national security policy and military strategy. GHE activities establish, reconstitute, maintain, or improve the capabilities or capacities of the PN's military or civilian health sector, or those of the DoD.[11]

DoD has been tasked to employ GHE to support a growing list of U.S. national security missions since the end of the Cold War, including stabilization, irregular warfare operations, and responding to weapon threats.[12] The list of missions has expanded to building global capacity to respond to outbreaks of infectious disease and contributing to international efforts, such as the Global Health Security Agenda.[13]

Although it is difficult to quantify the demand for GHE, the need for military medical personnel to engage with partner nations has clearly grown more acute as DoD has been called on to respond to the coronavirus disease 2019 (COVID-19) pandemic while meeting evolving strategic competition challenges. Working with allies and partners to improve their medical capabilities and degree of interoperability with the United States has become increasingly necessary to ensure that U.S. forces remain healthy and ready to conduct contingency operations, including a potential conflict with a near-peer adversary. Such potential conflicts would create

---

[11] DoD Instruction 2000.30, *Global Health Engagement (GHE) Activities*, U.S. Department of Defense, July 12, 2017, p. 19.

[12] GHE has become a component of a series of U.S. missions, including building partner capacity for stabilization operations (DoD Directive 3000.05, *Stabilization*, U.S. Department of Defense, December 13, 2018), supporting unconventional warfare for irregular warfare operations (DoD Directive 3000.07, *Irregular Warfare (IW)*, U.S. Department of Defense, Incorporating Change 1, May 12, 2017), addressing biological threats under the Cooperative Threat Reduction program (DoD Directive 2060.02, *DoD Countering Weapons of Mass Destruction (WMD) Policy*, U.S. Department of Defense, January 27, 2017), conducting foreign disaster relief missions (DoD Directive 5100.46, *Foreign Disaster Relief (FDR)*, U.S. Department of Defense, Incorporating Change 1, July 28, 2017), engaging in Humanitarian and Civic Assistance (HCA) during military operations (DoD Instruction 2205.02, *Humanitarian and Civic Assistance (HCA) Activities*, U.S. Department of Defense, Incorporating Change 1, May 22, 2017), and building partner capacity for force health protection (DoD Instruction 6200.04, *Force Health Protection (FHP)*, U.S. Department of Defense, April 23, 2007). See DoD Instruction 2000.30 (2017).

[13] DoD is among the U.S. government agencies that supports the Global Health Security Agenda, a U.S.-led partnership of over 70 nations designed to build global capacity to prevent, detect, and respond to infectious diseases (Global Health Security Agenda, "About the GHSA," webpage, undated). President Joe Biden reaffirmed U.S. commitment to the Global Health Security Agenda at the G7 meeting in 2021.

significantly higher demands for casualty care and a greater need to rely on U.S. allies and partners for medical support because of the tyranny of distance and high demand for expeditionary medical support.[14] Moreover, DoD's emphasis on agile combat employment across the services and the associated requirement for more-distributed basing will require force health protection across a wider range of locations. In this report, we takes the first step toward identifying (1) GHE priorities for meeting geographic combatant command (GCC) objectives and (2) the implications that GHE funding has on meeting GCC requirements (particularly, requirements related to U.S. force protection and medical readiness).

To date, funding for GHE activities has come from a multitude of sources, none of which provide sustained multiyear support, which a 2018 capabilities-based assessment (CBA) stated was critical to achieving GCC long-term objectives.[15] Given the CBA's finding, which was confirmed by the comments of the military medical personnel we interviewed, we assume that this lack of consistent funding has limited the ability of the medical community to develop partner-nation medical capacity and the interoperable medical capabilities necessary to ensure U.S. medical readiness and force protection requirements to meet GCC objectives.

In this introductory chapter, we describe the range of GHE activities and stakeholders and the complexity and limitations of current funding mechanisms. We then outline our research approach for addressing these funding challenges before summarizing the contents of the rest of this report.

GHE Activities and Stakeholders Have Expanded

The extent of DoD's engagement in global health over the past two decades has become so diverse and varied that GHE activities have become difficult to identify or quantify. GHE has expanded beyond a tool for improving the health and safety of U.S. warfighters and expanding medical readiness to encompass objectives related to (1) building trust and deepening professional medical relationships with partner nations and (2) advancing U.S. national security objectives more broadly.[16] According to DoD Instruction 2000.30, GHE may support any national security objectives related to

- fostering collaboration with military, government, or civil society

---

[14] The demands of large-scale combat operations and requirements for disbursed operations could also drive shortfalls in the provision of medical logistics and sustainment support. Partner nations could be critical to securing medical supplies, patient transport, and possibly even treatment for troops wounded in combat. For information on the future demands for casualty care in a potential conflict with near-peer adversaries and the relevance of GHE in preparing for these operations, see Brent Thomas, *Preparing for the Future of Combat Casualty Care: Opportunities to Refine the Military Health System's Alignment with the National Defense Strategy*, RAND Corporation, RR-A713-1, 2021, p. 49.

[15] DoD, *Global Health Engagement (GHE) Capabilities-Based Assessment (CBA) Study*, July 23, 2018, Not available to the general public.

[16] DoD, Military Health System, "Global Health Engagement," webpage, undated-b.

- engaging with partners to achieve security cooperation objectives
- enhancing the readiness of DoD medical forces and sustainably improving the operational skills of partner-nation personnel
- improving interoperability in coalition, bilateral, or multinational activities
- promoting stability and security
- establishing or maintaining a level of health and a state of preparedness conducive to healthy human and animal populations, which bolsters the civilian population's confidence in partner-nation governance.[17]

As the military has been called on to pursue a wider range of national security objectives through its health engagements, the spectrum of activities that fall under the framework of GHE has expanded. Figure 1.1 provides the version of the GHE conceptual framework that is featured in DoD Instruction 2000.30, which depicts GHE falling into four broad overlapping areas:

1. force health protection
2. humanitarian assistance and disaster relief
3. nuclear, chemical, and biological defense programs
4. building partner capacity and interoperability.[18]

Within each of these categories, there is a long list of building partnership capacity, exercises, and education and training efforts.

---

[17] DoD Instruction 2000.30, 2017, p. 3.

[18] DoD Instruction 2000.30, 2017.

Figure 1.1. Spectrum of DoD GHE Activities

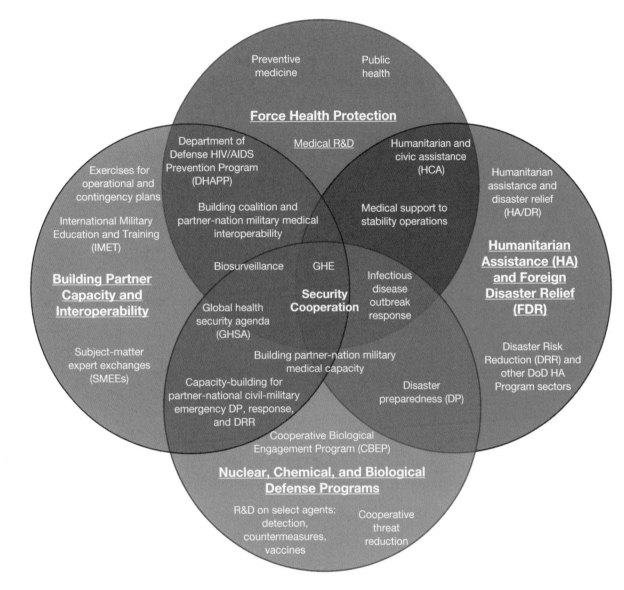

SOURCE: Adapted from Uniformed Services University, "Department of Defense Global Health Engagement," briefing, undated; and DoD Instruction 2000.30, 2017, p. 4.
NOTE: R&D = research and development.

A vast number of organizations and stakeholders—including the Office of the Secretary of Defense and Joint Chiefs of Staff, all of the functional and geographic commands and military departments, and several DoD field agencies—oversee, plan, and conduct these wide-ranging activities. In a 2012 review of DoD's role in global health, Kaiser Family Foundation researchers identified myriad DoD organizations engaged in GHE.[19] Both the GCC command surgeons' offices and the command surgeons' offices within distinct service component commands play a

---

[19] Josh Michaud, Kellie Moss, and Jen Kates, *The U.S. Department of Defense and Global Health: Technical Volume*, Kaiser Family Foundation, September 2012.

role in planning and conducting activities, as do National Guard units through the State Partnership Program (SPP). Command surgeons' offices at U.S. Special Operations Command (SOCOM) and the Theater Special Operations Commands are also engaged in GHE activities, as are the U.S. Strategic Command and U.S. Transportation Command.

Each of the services also has a role in deploying military medical capabilities to conduct activities and educate and train both U.S. and partner military forces in issues related to global health (including targeted programs, such as the Defense Institute for Medical Operations). Medical research labs led by the services engage with partner nations, and regional centers and organizations such as the Center for Excellence in Disaster Management and Humanitarian Assistance in the U.S. Indo-Pacific Command (INDOPACOM) provide health-related courses to U.S. forces and partner militaries alike. Moreover, DoD's Defense Threat Reduction Agency (DTRA) has the lead on conducting GHE activities related to deliberate biological and chemical threats through its Cooperative Threat Reduction program. The Defense Security Cooperation Agency (DSCA) oversees most humanitarian assistance and disaster relief programs and building partner capacity (BPC) efforts, and the Uniformed Services University of the Health Sciences (USUHS) conducts global health education programs.

This diversity of stakeholders within the DoD community, as well as the over 85 organizations within the interagency community involved in global health security, has enabled opportunity for engagement across all aspects of global health.[20] However, it also makes it difficult to derive a common understanding of GHE and its purpose in supporting U.S. national security objectives. The various perspectives on global health have often prevented health engagements from being effectively prioritized in DoD capability planning.[21] Indeed, this expansive list of activities and stakeholders has led to a lack of common understanding of GHE and its application to U.S. national security objectives. It has also made it difficult to assess or evaluate the impact of GHE activities.

Medical planners within the GCCs often have difficulty demonstrating how GHE activities support theater campaign plans or applying an ends-ways-means framework to partner-nation engagement.[22] In other words, GHE may not be clearly defined as a "way" to achieve theater

---

[20] A 2012 Kaiser Family Foundation report identified an expansive list of DoD organizations involved in GHE activities, as well as 85 coordinating interagency partners. See Michaud, Moss, and Kates (2012).

[21] The U.S. government organizations and agencies engaged in the Global Health Security Agenda includes the Departments of Defense, State, Justice, Agriculture, Health and Human Services, Treasury, Labor, and Homeland Security, as well as the Office of Management and Budget, Office of the Director of National Intelligence, U.S. Agency for International Development, Environmental Protection Agency, Centers for Disease Control and Prevention, Office of Science and Technology Policy, National Institutes of Health, National Institute of Allergy and Infectious Diseases, and other agencies that the council determines appropriate (U.S. House of Representatives, Global Health Security Act of 2021, Bill 391, July 12, 2021).

[22] Arthur Lykke, Jr., developed the strategic framework of ends, ways, and means that has been used widely by the U.S. Army. This theory of strategy is often depicted mathematically as strategy = ends + ways + means, where "Strategy equals Ends (objectives towards which one strives) plus Ways (courses of action) plus Means (instruments

objectives or "ends" that enable strategy and lacks the connection to associated resources or "means" by which the ends can be achieved. Without a direct connection to theater plans, DoD's engagement in global health activities may be viewed as broadly beneficial but not critical to meeting U.S. strategic goals.

This broad perspective on GHE has contributed to a disjointed approach toward the funding. GHE activities are supported by a wide range of disparate funding mechanisms, for which the development of medical support capabilities is considered to be an ancillary objective. Although there are many potential funding sources for engaging with partners on global health issues, none are dedicated to building partner medical capacity or developing interoperable medical capabilities that could be needed to support U.S. operations. The complex patchwork of funding mechanisms has posed significant challenges for the implementation and sustainment of GHE activities and has complicated the work of security cooperation professionals. It has also led to missed opportunities when it comes to integrating GHE activities in support of operational objectives across the GCCs.

A CBA of GHE conducted in 2018 and sponsored by the Deputy Assistant Secretary of Defense (DASD) for Health Readiness Policy and Oversight examined DoD's ability to conduct GHE activities in support of combatant commanders' objectives. The CBA identified shortfalls related to an inadequate awareness and understanding of GHE as a tool for achieving combatant command theater objectives, a lack of a joint professional cadre of global health specialists with a common standard of competencies, and inadequate incorporation of GHE into professional educational venues. The assessment also identified a need to better capture, track, and monitor execution of GHE activities and assess the effectiveness of GHE activities, noting that DoD has insufficient means to analyze the status of partner-nation health systems and assistance needs. In addition, the CBA highlighted DoD's lack of funding to support and sustain GHE priority activities in support of long-term objectives.[23]

Following the CBA, a Joint Requirements Oversight Council endorsed a DOTmLPF-P[24] Change Recommendation with 15 recommendations intended to address the shortfalls that limit effective and efficient GHE support to combatant command theater campaign plans.[25] Seven of the 15 actions require additional, independent research. The Office of the Assistant Secretary of Defense (OASD) for Health Affairs asked RAND researchers to support all seven of these actions to help DoD synchronize GHE training and education, use the most efficient technology

---

by which some end can be achieved)" (Arthur F. Lykke, Jr., "A Methodology for Developing a Military Strategy," in Arthur F. Lykke, Jr., ed., *Military Strategy: Theory and Application*, U.S. Army War College, 1993, p. 3).

[23] DoD, 2018.

[24] DOTmLPF-P stands for Doctrine, Organization, Training, materiel, Leadership and education, Personnel, Facilities, and Policy.

[25] Paul Selva, Vice Chairman of the Joint Chiefs of Staff, "DOTmLPF-P Change Recommendation for Global Health Engagement," memorandum, JROCM 008-19, February 25, 2019.

platforms, and orchestrate funding mechanisms to enable long-term GHE capability development.[26]

Research Task and Approach

This report presents the results of our research on the task related to funding, which came about as result of the CBA's finding that DoD lacked a funding mechanism that supports long-term GHE activities.[27] Specifically, our task was to identify funding sources that support GHE activities and consider the implications of multiyear funding. This included identifying funding sources that can be used to support multiyear GHE activities and exploring the feasibility of establishing GHE as a program of record.[28]

To conduct this task, we began by looking at the various funding mechanisms that are currently being used to support global health–related activities (an overview of current funding mechanisms can be found in Appendix A). We then sought to identify current gaps in funding by asking medical planners across the GCCs about their priorities for conducting GHE activities and how these activities supported theater objectives. Next, we asked GHE stakeholders about their current activities, how they funded these activities, and what obstacles they faced in meeting their objectives. In this way, we intended to gain a better understanding of GHE challenges and whether a new funding mechanism might be required. With this knowledge, we sought to outline what a new funding mechanism might look like to better support GCC objectives.

---

[26] These seven recommendations are to

- conduct a feasibility study on the development of a joint GHE Intellipedia-like site
- review, revise, and (if necessary) develop GHE-related training modules
- conduct a technology survey to identify potential commercial off-the-shelf solutions to identify, collect, synthesize, analyze, and report GHE data
- review, revise, and (if necessary) develop GHE-related education courses across DoD to incorporate key principles outlined by DoD Instruction 2000.30
- review and, as appropriate, revise medical planner and other relevant courses to incorporate GHE planning requirements
- review and, as appropriate, incorporate pertinent curriculum material into Joint Professional Military Education core security cooperation curricula
- conduct a pilot study to ascertain whether multiyear funding and/or the establishment of GHE as a program of record to align multiple funding streams will help GHE activities advance the combatant commands' Theater Campaign Plans.

[27] The two other reports in this series are Jefferson P. Marquis, Trupti Brahmbhatt, Aaron Clark-Ginsberg, Victoria M. Smith, and David E. Thaler, *Educating and Training the Department of Defense Workforce for Global Health Engagement to Support the Geographic Combatant Commands*, RAND Corporation, RR-A1357-1, 2023; and Padmaja Vedula, Trupti Brahmbhatt, Jonathan Tran, and Chandler Sachs, *Assessing Technology Platforms for Global Health Engagement to Support Integration of Efforts Across Geographic Combatant Commands*, RAND Corporation, RR-A1357-3, 2023.

[28] The term *program of record* refers to a DoD program that is recorded in the current Future Years Defense Program and is identified as a line item in the DoD annual budget. The term most commonly refers to programs and systems in the DoD acquisition process that are funded by the national defense authorization act (DoD, *Non-Program of Record U.S. Industry Handbook*, July 2020, p. 5).

Thus, to identify the funding sources supporting GHE activities and the potential implications for obtaining more-consistent support for long-term GHE efforts, we began by addressing the following four key research questions regarding the purpose of GHE:

- How does GHE support theater plans?
- What type of GHE activities are being conducted?
- What are the primary funding sources used to support GHE activities?
- What challenges do current GHE funding mechanisms pose?

Then, to consider the feasibility of (1) establishing GHE as a program of record or (2) a dedicated funding source, we addressed two additional research questions:

- In what areas is GHE funding needed to meet theater objectives?
- What types of funds could better meet U.S. objectives or support GCC efforts to a greater extent?

We began with a review of the literature on GHE programs and funding sources, including relevant laws, DoD instructions, and policies associated with GHE and security cooperation, as well as databases, academic journal articles, and military medical journals. However, because of the lack of comprehensive data or scholarship on GHE activity, we relied heavily on discussions with U.S. defense officials for our analysis. We then followed up on these discussions with expert group discussions to validate our findings.

We held a series of semistructured discussions with more than 75 GHE stakeholders from across the command surgeons' offices and five GCCs—U.S. Africa Command (AFRICOM), U.S. Central Command (CENTCOM), U.S. European Command (EUCOM), INDOPACOM, and U.S. Southern Command (SOUTHCOM)[29]—as well as across their respective air components: U.S. Air Forces Africa (AFAFRICA), U.S. Air Forces Central (AFCENT), U.S. Air Forces Europe (USAFE), U.S. Air Forces Pacific (PACAF), and U.S. Air Forces Southern (AFSOUTH). Participants in these discussions included both command surgeons and GHE personnel.

We then did a deeper dive into INDOPACOM, for which we spoke with the combatant command surgeon and PACAF surgeon and their staff, as well as representatives from each of the other service components. This included U.S. Army Pacific (USARPAC), U.S. Pacific Fleet (PACFLT), and U.S. Marine Corps Forces, Pacific (MARFORPAC). Because of its growing strategic importance in U.S. defense policy, INDOPACOM became the subject of a deeper analysis of GHE priorities, activities, and funding.

In addition to the GCCs and component commands, we spoke to security cooperation planners within DSCA, as well as representatives from DTRA and the Center for Excellence in Disaster Management and Humanitarian Assistance in INDOPACOM. We also engaged with

---

[29] Although we spoke with an official in the command surgeon in the sixth GCC (U.S. Northern Command), the official indicated that the office engages in a limited number of GHE activities and does not face any funding challenges in terms of conducting those activities.

command surgeons at U.S. Transportation Command and SOCOM, as well as medical and security cooperation officers in two SOCOM component commands—the Air Force Special Operations Command and the Army Special Operations Command—and one theater special operations command.[30]

We asked each discussion participant to address our key research questions. We asked them the following:

- What are your GHE priorities? How does GHE support your theater plans?
- What types of GHE activities do you currently conduct?
- What primary funding sources do you use?
- What challenges do you face in obtaining funding?
- Are there other types of funds that could better meet U.S. objectives?

A complete list of the organizations that participated in discussions and a sample discussion protocol can be found in Appendixes C and D, respectively. Subject-matter experts on the research team reviewed each of the interview notes separately, conducting independent findings that were then validated. We used this combined analysis to compile a list of each GCC's GHE priorities and outlined the distinct ways in which each priority supports the operational needs of the respective combatant command. We also identified commonalities and differences across primary global health–related activities in each GCC, the funding sources they relied on most, and the challenges that each GCC faces in implementing GHE activities.

During the next stage of our research, we conducted two 90-minute virtual group discussions with members of the Joint Staff and representatives from each of the GCCs, the Office of the Secretary of Defense, and DSCA. The discussions also included a representative from the Office of the Secretary of Defense Comptroller's office and a member of the office's legal team and generally helped to validate our findings and recognize areas that required additional research.

There were several limitations to our study. First, although we engaged with a significant number of GHE stakeholders, we were not able to cover the full range of organizations that carry out or are otherwise involved in GHE. By focusing on the GCCs and their components, we did not track the GHE activities conducted by the services though professional military education (e.g., International Military Education and Training [IMET] courses by the Defense Institute for Medical Operations, medical research and development [through service labs], or disease surveillance activities undertaken by DTRA under the Cooperative Threat Reduction program). We also did not capture funding challenges associated with these programs and activities.

Second, we conducted our study during the COVID-19 pandemic, which prevented us from conducting in-person discussions and notably affected the data that we received on GHE

---

[30] All interviews were conducted on a non-attributional basis; RAND's Human Subjects Protection Committee determined the study did not require the protection of human subjects per DoD Instruction 3216.02, *Protection of Human Subjects and Adherence to Ethical Standards in DoD-Conducted and -Supported Research*, U.S. Department of Defense, April 15, 2020.

activities. The scope of GHE programs and activities was also severely constrained during 2020 and 2021 because U.S. defense health officials and other key stakeholders were unable to travel to engage in previously scheduled activities with partner nations; these stakeholders were also consumed by responding to the immediate effects of the pandemic on U.S. forces. Because of rapid staff turnover, some of the officials we spoke with had limited experience or activity data from the pre-pandemic era. Nevertheless, we were able to conduct discussions with many personnel who had been engaged in GHE activities in their previous positions and were thus able to provide a longer-term perspective.

Interestingly, we found that the COVID-19 pandemic brought the need for GHE into greater focus because it served to highlight the importance of addressing public health concerns, both as a means of ensuring U.S. force protection and medical readiness and as a means of developing closer relationships with partner nations.

Organization of This Report

The rest of this report is organized as follows. In Chapter Two, we begin by outlining the GHE priorities and activities in each of the five major GCCs and identifying some of the commonalities and differences among the regions. Chapter Three provides an overview of the current funding sources that the GCCs use to fund GHE activities, the challenges that personnel across the GCCs have faced in identifying and accessing funding for GHE activities, and the difficulties they face in planning activities and in building partner-nation capabilities and capacity. In Chapter Four, we include key findings and recommendations and offer various courses of action to provide more-consistent funding for GHE to meet GCC operational requirements. We consider options for better leveraging existing funds and for establishing a new program of record and lay out the advantages and disadvantages of each funding option.

Finally, we provide more-detailed information about our findings and research methods in the appendixes. Appendix A provides a list and explanation of the primary GHE-related security cooperation funding sources. Appendix B provides detailed information on GCC priorities and activities, as well as a list of the primary GHE activities conducted by each of the components in INDOPACOM. Appendixes C and D provide the list of organizations that we engaged and the discussion protocol.

Chapter 2. Global Health Engagement Priorities and Activities

The first step in determining the need for GHE funding is to consider current GHE priorities. We sought to answer this question by asking senior leaders in the medical community and personnel within each of the command surgeons' offices about their GHE priorities. We asked them to describe the types of GHE capabilities that they were seeking to develop and how GHE priorities support their respective combatant command's objectives. We found that answers to these questions varied. GHE priorities and the emphasis on GHE activities differ by combatant command. Moreover, we found that, in many cases, GHE activities are planned from the "bottom up" to take advantage of opportunities as they arise, making it difficult to align GHE activities to a particular theater's objectives or plan or to establish a clear link between the ends, ways, and means to achieve overarching theater strategies.[31]

In this chapter, we provide an overview of GHE priorities in each of the five GCCs included in our study: INDOPACOM, CENTCOM, EUCOM, AFRICOM, and SOUTHCOM.[32] We then consider how these priorities lead to different types of GHE activities, recognizing that GHE objectives are not always clearly defined and that GHE activities do not always align directly with these objectives or their respective theater plans. It is important to note that we capture service component activities within each of their respective combatant commands and do not address the distinct differences in the ways each component prioritizes and conducts its activities, nor do we address the way in which these activities are coordinated. A more complete list of activities of each service component is included in Appendix B. The issue of coordinating activities across GCCs is important but is beyond the scope of our analysis.

We start with an analysis of GHE in the Indo-Pacific region (because it was the focus of our in-depth analysis), then look at the other four GCCs in comparison. Finally, we look at common themes in capability and capacity development that extend beyond regional objectives.

GHE Priorities Vary Across GCCs

GHE priorities in INDOPACOM are focused on improving relationships with allies and partners and, increasingly, on developing interoperable medical capabilities. Historically, medical outreach and humanitarian assistance and disaster response efforts, such as those undertaken by U.S. Navy hospital ships (e.g., USNS Mercy), have been viewed by the medical community as a means of achieving greater access and influence in critical regions where the

---

[31] Discussions with U.S. defense officials, November 23, 2020, and January 25, 2021.

[32] U.S. Northern Command was not included in our study.

United States otherwise has limited presence.[33] GHE strategy has continued to evolve to focus on achieving more-favorable regional perceptions of the United States, attracting partners and sustaining relationships in the region, decreasing health security risks in the region, and integrating health capabilities within and across partner countries to enhance U.S. posture and deterrence.[34]

According to U.S. defense officials, as more attention has been placed on strategic competition against China, medical planners have become more concerned about improving U.S. posture and readiness in the Indo-Pacific region: specifically, on building interoperable medical capabilities to strengthen response to contingencies.[35] Although INDOPACOM's 2020 Health Theater Security Cooperation Strategy points to a wide range of goals related to improving relationships and humanitarian efforts, it explicitly states that global health should serve as a strategic enabler that improves readiness and benefits campaign plan objectives.[36] Thus, the INDOPACOM GHE strategy appears to focus on both developing more-interoperable regional military medical capabilities and increasing access to support contingencies.

GHE priorities outlined by INDOPACOM component commands reflect a similar trend. The USARPAC Surgeon's Office views health engagements as a means of assuring allies, gaining access, and generating mutual readiness. USARPAC GHE plans emphasize the importance of sharing information and coordinating activities with partner-nation military medical personnel to achieve interoperability to facilitate joint and combined operational processes.[37] As of fiscal year 2021, USARPAC had developed a series of Five-Year Country Health Engagement Plans for ten countries in the region.[38] These plans relate partner capability and capacity objectives to U.S. national security policy and military strategies but do not specifically mention GCC theater plans.

We found that PACFLT, MARFORPAC, and PACAF have specifically focused their GHE priorities on supporting the medical readiness of U.S. forces and the readiness of forces across the theater.[39] MARFORPAC's priorities are similar to PACFLT's, given that many of its activities are nested under PACFLT initiatives.

---

[33] Medical and humanitarian missions to the Pacific island states are often cited as efforts intended to increase U.S. influence (discussion with U.S. defense official, January 22, 2021).

[34] Unpublished 2020 GHE strategy information provided to the authors by INDOPACOM.

[35] Discussion with U.S. defense officials, November 12, 2020, and April 29, 2021.

[36] Unpublished 2020 GHE strategy information provided to the authors by INDOPACOM and discussion with U.S. defense officials, January 7, 2021.

[37] USARPAC Surgeon's Office, "Health Theater Security Cooperation/Global Health Engagement Deep Dive," briefing, September 2020.

[38] USARPAC completed country plans for Bangladesh, Mongolia, Nepal, Palau, Sri Lanka, Thailand, Vietnam, Indonesia, the Philippines, and India.

[39] Discussion with U.S. defense official, February 26, 2021.

PACAF GHE priorities have focused on building the capabilities of partners for humanitarian assistance and disaster response—specifically, as they pertain to aeromedical evacuation—which is helpful in force health protection and strategic competition objectives.[40] Thus, medical planners from each of the components indicated that these activities were intended not only to increase U.S. access and influence but also to gain more regional capability to support potential contingencies. However, neither INDOPACOM nor the components appear to directly link GHE to the need to respond to large-scale casualties in a potential contingency as part of efforts to "build regional resilience to 21st century transnational threats" described in the U.S. Indo-Pacific strategy.[41]

GHE priorities in EUCOM are somewhat different from those in INDOPACOM because they have been more consistently focused on meeting operational requirements.[42] EUCOM GHE personnel indicated that GHE priorities have long centered on improving partner-nation capability to contribute to operations in Afghanistan and, since 2014, on a potential military conflict in Europe.[43] As one official noted, "we are investing in the medical capabilities of our partners in Eastern Europe because we believe that if a partner nation or new North Atlantic Treaty Organization (NATO) partner nation has such a capability, then [U.S. forces] will not have to deploy our medics and we can utilize partner-nation capabilities to support our troops."[44] These priorities align with EUCOM plans to improve U.S. posture and presence in Europe by focusing on developing interoperable military medical capabilities among countries in the former Soviet Union to support combined NATO operations. However, officials indicated that GHE priorities did not include efforts to enhance interoperability with Western European nations or broader efforts to improve medical capabilities across the region in the event of a conflict.[45]

In the CENTCOM region, GHE priorities have been directed toward improving medical capabilities to support current operations. GHE has been used as a vehicle for building security partnerships in countries in Central Asia, similar to the way it has been used to open doors in the Indo-Pacific region. However, for the most part, GHE has been used to promote partner military medical readiness and interoperability.[46] As one DoD official noted, "due to ongoing operations, generating military medical readiness is particularly important in the AOR [area of responsibility]."[47] Notably, developing military medical capabilities to U.S. standards is important for many partner nations and for CENTCOM planners to provide better support for

[40] Discussions with U.S. defense officials, February 2021 and March 1, 4, and 18, 2021.

[41] The White House, *Indo-Pacific Strategy of the United States*, February 2022, p. 14.

[42] Discussions with U.S. defense officials, August 11, 2020, and March 24, 2021.

[43] Discussion with DoD officials, March 24, 2021.

[44] Discussion with DoD officials, March 24, 2021.

[45] Discussion with DoD officials, August 11, 2020.

[46] Discussions with DoD officials, March 9, 2021.

[47] Discussions with DoD officials, March 9, 2021.

U.S. forces across the Middle East and Central Asia. Given CENTCOM's focus on ongoing conflicts in the Middle East and Central Asia, the command prioritizes the development of tactical capability and military medical readiness for current operations. Still, GHE activities are not presented as contributing directly to theater military medical readiness or broader theater strategy.[48]

GHE priorities in AFRICOM are primarily focused on improving regional stability by enabling partners to ensure the health of their forces and respond to outbreaks of infectious disease.[49] GHE is also seen as a means of applying soft power in the region relative to other strategic competitors.[50] Medical personnel in AFRICOM noted that medical missions are particularly advantageous for achieving access and influence. By providing support to health sectors of otherwise underdeveloped countries, "we get access and are able to be [in locations] where [local populations] may not want combat [troops]."[51] Such access is viewed as increasingly important in meeting new theater priorities related to enabling global operations. Moreover, officials indicated that GHE activities are also necessary to sustain the health and protection of U.S. forces involved in ongoing counterterrorism operations or future small-scale contingency operations in the region.[52] Thus, GHE strategy is focused not only on building military medical capacity and disease response to improve stability but also on protecting U.S. forces.

SOUTHCOM's GHE is primarily focused on building regional medical response capabilities and improving the public health sectors of partner countries.[53] Medical planners stressed that military medical engagements are particularly valuable when it comes to building local partnerships and ensuring that the United States remains the primary provider of military medical training and capacity-building to regional partners.[54] DoD officials emphasized that GHE activities also tie into SOUTHCOM's objectives related to strategic competition by enabling closer engagement with U.S. allies and partners. Moreover, GHE has increasingly been seen as a means of ensuring force protection and improving force readiness in the region by providing training opportunities for U.S. forces.[55] SOUTHCOM's vision for GHE is to improve public health and U.S. medical readiness through coordinated capacity-building health engagement

---

[48] Discussions with U.S. defense official, March 2, 2021.

[49] AFRICOM, "AFRICOM'S Health Engagements," briefing, September 4, 2019, Not available to the general public.

[50] AFRICOM, 2019.

[51] Discussion with DoD officials, January 26, 2021.

[52] Discussions with U.S. defense officials, January 14, 2021; and AFRICOM, 2019.

[53] Discussion with DoD official, March 25, 2021.

[54] Discussion with DoD official, March 4, 2021.

[55] SOUTHCOM, "A Partnership Approach to Global Health Engagements," briefing, undated, Not available to the general public.

efforts.[56] However, this vision was not directly tied to combatant command plans in a way that demonstrated how GHE contributed to strategic objectives. Our analysis of GHE priorities across GCCs indicated that GHE strategies are broadly stated, covering a wide range of objectives. Yet, they are focused differently according to theater demands in each region. In EUCOM and CENTCOM, where there are ongoing or future operations, there is an emphasis on building partner-nation capabilities to support U.S. forces. In AFRICOM and SOUTHCOM, there is more of a focus on partner-nation capacity-building and disease surveillance. And in INDOPACOM, there is a combination of GHE priorities focused on developing partner-nation capabilities and interoperability that could be used in the event of a contingency and on developing partner-nation capacity for addressing health threats. As we discuss in more detail in the next section, these distinctions are important to understand the type of activities that each GCC is interested in building to support strategic requirements. The commonalities across GCCs in seeking to address issues related to force protection and medical readiness may help to demonstrate how GHE contributes to theater strategy and may ultimately be important in regard to how these activities are prioritized and funded.

GCC GHE Activities Vary According to Theater Priorities

The types of GHE activities that each GCC has pursued and would like to pursue have varied in relation to their priorities. In this section, we provide an overview of the major activities outlined by the command surgeons' offices over roughly a four-year period, from 2018 to 2021.[57] We note how the GCCs' GHE priorities have shaped their activities during this time frame and the type of activities that they would like to engage in the future to meet evolving strategic priorities.

INDOPACOM GHE Activities Focus on Public Health Outreach, Disease Prevention and Surveillance, and Increasingly on Trauma Care and Casualty Evacuation

As we note above, GHE priorities in the Indo-Pacific have historically focused on expanding U.S. access and influence, leading to significant efforts focused on medical outreach and humanitarian and disaster response in countries where the United States does not maintain close ties. Military medical activities related to disease surveillance and preventive medicine have continued to be important, particularly in light of the COVID-19 pandemic and the ensuing need for more actions focusing on force health protection within U.S. and partner-nation forces.[58]

---

[56] SOUTHCOM, undated.

[57] Recognizing that many activities were canceled or postponed in 2020 and 2021 because of the COVID-19 pandemic, we asked about activities during the previous two years.

[58] Discussion with defense personnel, February 18, 2021.

At the same time, as concerns have grown over a potential conflict in the region, demand for GHE activities that can improve partner nations' medical capabilities and interoperability with the United States has also increased. Across the service components in INDOPACOM, DoD officials pointed to what they see as a growing demand for engagements and training exercises aimed at improving partner nations' expeditionary medicine and trauma care capabilities, as well as their ability to conduct medical evacuation (MEDEVAC) and casualty evacuation (CASEVAC). These efforts were noted to be important to improving medical readiness for a potential contingency in the region.

In fiscal year 2021, INDOPACOM's Army component, USARPAC, planned to conduct GHE activities in ten countries, primarily in South and Southeast Asia.[59] These activities included subject-matter expert exchanges in bio-preparedness for public health and force health protection, as well as trauma and triage patient care and MEDEVAC training during exercises.[60] Although many in-person training events were canceled because of the COVID-19 pandemic, planners noted they intend to focus on trauma care and ground and rotary-wing evacuation training in the future. They indicated that USARPAC was specifically seeking to engage with one more-capable country by focusing on trauma care in austere and high-altitude environments.[61] Other engagements conducted under the National Guard SPP were also planned to increase bilateral and multilateral interoperability for peacekeeping operations and crisis response.[62]

PACAF officials described plans for U.S. airmen to continue to be involved in annual engagements, such as PACIFIC ANGEL, which provides medical care, engineering assistance, and subject-matter expert expertise in such countries as Bangladesh, Mongolia, and Papua New Guinea.[63] At the same time, they noted that greater emphasis is being placed on trilateral exercises with close U.S. allies, such as Australia and Japan, in aeromedical evacuation and mass casualty field training exercises.[64] Among the more-capable partner nations, PACAF saw not only a growing need for medical readiness but also an increasing interest among partner air

---

[59] Many of the activities planned for fiscal year 2021 were postponed or canceled because of the COVID-19 pandemic.

[60] Trauma training was scheduled to occur during the BALIKATAN exercises, for example (USARPAC, "FY21 Health Security Cooperation/Global Health Engagement OAIs," undated, Not available to the general public).

[61] USARPAC Surgeon's Office, 2020.

[62] Discussion with U.S. defense officials, March 2021.

[63] Mikaley Kline, "Pacific Angel Provides Aid, Builds Partnerships Throughout Indo-Pacific Communities," U.S. Indo-Pacific Command, October 1, 2019.

[64] Major exercises with more-capable U.S. partners include COPE NORTH, which involved a multilateral aeromedical evacuation exercise in 2018 and mass casualty field training in 2020 (discussion with U.S. defense official, March 1, 2021; Gregory Nash, "Multinational Medics, Civilian First Responders 'Save Lives' at Exercise Cope North 2020," U.S. Air Force, March 2, 2020; and Juan Torres Chardon, "Crews Provide Aeromedical Evacuation Capabilities in Cope North Exercise," U.S. Department of Defense, February 28, 2018).

forces to improve their CASEVAC and MEDEVAC capabilities and interoperability with the United States.[65]

Similarly, medical personnel in PACFLT indicated that they continued to engage in the Pacific Partnership annual military exercise to develop partner-nation evacuation capabilities and tactics, and they were planning to conduct more trauma and critical care training activities designed to increase interoperability with partner nations.[66] They also noted that they were particularly focused on *building shipboard medical capability among partner militaries, indicating that they would like to conduct more military-to-military* rather than military-to-civilian activities. Medical planners indicated that military-to-military activities aligned more closely with their desire to engage with partners in Oceania and throughout the region strategically to enhance the U.S. Navy's medical readiness and resiliency. Global health personnel at MARFORPAC also indicated that they focus on military-to-military engagements for exercises (e.g., BALIKATAN and COBRA GOLD) and partner capacity-building events with select partners, such as Thailand's Marine Corps. The 3rd Marine Expeditionary Force provides some subject-matter expert exchanges through the Pacific Partnership program but is most interested in conducting tactical military training, with such countries as Thailand, Malaysia, and Vietnam.[67] Medical planners we spoke with across the four component commands in INDOPACOM expressed a common desire to expand their engagement in military-to-military activities to increase partner-nation capacity and U.S. force protection and medical readiness.

EUCOM GHE Activities Focus on Expeditionary Medical Care and Improving Interoperability of Medical Capabilities

GHE planners in EUCOM and CENTCOM have placed a greater emphasis on conducting military-to-military activities. In Europe and the Middle East, where there is a greater focus on operational and contingency planning, most activities relate to expeditionary medical and trauma care and improving interoperability of medical capabilities with partner militaries.

EUCOM GHE activities involve visits and exchanges aimed at enabling partner forces to develop Role 1 and Role 2 and patient movement capabilities, as well medical logistics.[68] Much of this activity is focused on countries in Eastern Europe.[69] For many countries, this activity

---

[65] Discussion with U.S. defense official, February 18, 2021.

[66] Discussions with DoD officials, February 26, 2021.

[67] Discussion with U.S. defense official, March 1, 2021.

[68] Role 1 medical support includes capabilities for providing first aid, immediate lifesaving measures, and triage. Role 2 medical support includes advanced trauma management and emergency medical treatment (NATO, *NATO Logistics Handbook*, 3rd ed., October 1997, Ch. 16).

[69] As of 2021, EUCOM established health lines of activity for each of the following countries: Albania, Armenia, Azerbaijan, Bosnia and Herzegovina, Bulgaria, Croatia, Estonia, Georgia, Hungary, Kosovo, Latvia, Lithuania, Moldova, Montenegro, North Macedonia, Poland, Romania, Serbia, Slovenia, and Ukraine (EUCOM, *EUCOM*

involved helping establish standard operating procedures and conducting medical evaluations to ensure that Role 2 facilities meet NATO standards (even in some countries, such as Georgia, that are not NATO members).[70] GHE engagement in Poland has focused on developing the country's MEDEVAC capabilities to improve its interoperability with NATO through subject-matter expert exchanges and exercises.[71] In Southeast Europe, GHE activities are focused on the development of a Balkan Medical Task Force. This effort, which is conducted with assistance from Norway, is intended to build a deployable, rotational, multinational NATO Role 2 medical treatment facility in the region.[72] For Ukraine, EUCOM provided institutional capacity-building support to the Ministry of Health by providing an advisor to develop a rehabilitation agency for veterans that is similar to the Department of Veterans Affairs in the United States.[73]

Several other Eastern and Western European countries are engaged in GHE activities through exercises and key leader engagements on related topics but do not have a dedicated Health Line of Activity.[74] Medical planners noted that several of these countries (particularly, Denmark, the United Kingdom, and Italy) have expressed an *interest in working with the United States to develop their military medical capabilities and increase interoperability in the region.*[75]

U.S. Army Europe and Africa (USAREUR-AF), USAFE, the National Guard's SPP, the Defense Institute for Medical Operations, the NATO Center of Excellence for Military Medicine, and other entities are leading or participating in global health engagements throughout the theater. Medical planners at USAFE indicated that they are primarily engaged in helping partner nations certify their Role 1 and Role 2 medical treatment facilities, ensuring they are built according to NATO standards. USAFE personnel are also engaged in familiarization and exchange visits related to mental health, aerospace medicine, and aerial patient movement. Moreover, U.S. airmen participate in NATO medical readiness exercises, such as VIGOROUS WARRIOR, which includes 39 partner nations. Despite the COVID-19 restrictions in place in 2020 and 2021 that limited exercises and in-person visits, U.S. defense officials indicated that

---

Combatant Command Campaign Plan 2020: Global Health Engagement, 2021, Appendix 10 to Annex Q, Not available to the general public).

[70] Discussions with DoD personnel, March 1, 2021.

[71] Discussions with DoD personnel, March 1, 2021; Rafal Mniedlo, "Allied Spirit Medical Evacuation (MEDEVAC) Training in Poland," U.S. Army Europe and Africa, June 6, 2020; and Armando A. Schwier-Morales, "USAFE Offers Knowledge to Polish Flying Doctors," Air Force Medical Service, December 7, 2015.

[72] EUCOM, *EUCOM Combatant Command Campaign Plan 2018: Health Security Cooperation*, May 15, 2018, Appendix 3 to Annex Q, Not available to the general public.

[73] Discussion with U.S. defense official, August 11, 2020.

[74] These countries include Austria, Belarus, Cyprus, the Czech Republic, Denmark, Finland, France, Germany, Greece, Italy, Malta, the Netherlands, Norway, Spain, Sweden, Turkey, and the United Kingdom.

[75] Discussions with DoD personnel, March 1, 2021.

partners expressed an increasing interest in developing interoperable air capabilities. This interest was particularly strong among more-capable European allies.[76]

CENTCOM GHE Activities Focus on Interoperable Trauma Care and Evacuation Capabilities

GHE activities in CENTCOM are similar to EUCOM in that they include the development of Role 1 and Role 2 capabilities; however, there is more emphasis on building interoperable trauma care and evacuation capabilities. CENTCOM is also focused on medical readiness, working specifically with more-capable partners, such as the United Arab Emirates (UAE) and Jordan. Several defense officials pointed to the development of a Trauma, Burn, and Rehabilitative Medicine program in Abu Dhabi, UAE, as one of CENTCOM's most significant GHE activities in recent years, which includes military trauma experts embedded with Emirati military personnel in a civilian medical facility.[77] In Jordan, medical personnel provide training and certification for a nationwide trauma center. AFCENT has supported Kazakhstan's military medical training center. In addition, AFCENT has worked with Jordan on trauma and aeromedical evacuation during multinational exercises, such as EAGER LION and BRIGHT STAR.[78] DoD officials noted that AFCENT and other CENTCOM medical personnel were engaged in the training of the Afghan National Security Forces (ANSF) through 2021, when U.S. forces withdrew from the country. ANSF training was focused on combat casualty management and developing Afghan capability for CASEVAC and MEDEVAC.[79] U.S. officials noted that other partners have expressed an interest in developing aeromedical evacuation, but they have not yet engaged in major advise and assist efforts outside Afghanistan. The officials emphasized that the primary objective of the United States and partner nations across the region was to develop more-interoperable medical care capabilities.[80]

---

[76] The VIGOROUS WARRIOR exercise was postponed during the pandemic. In 2022, it was conducted as a tabletop exercise (NATO Centre of Excellence for Military Medicine, "Vigorous Warrior," webpage, undated; and discussions with DoD personnel, March 1, 2021).

[77] Derek Licina and Jackson Taylor, "International Trauma Capacity Building Programs: Modernizing Capabilities, Enhancing Lethality, Supporting Alliances, Building Partnerships, and Implementing Reform," *Military Medicine*, Vol. 187, No. 7–8, July–August 2022.

[78] Discussions with U.S. defense officials, March 9, 2021.

[79] CENTCOM medical personnel were not involved in similar partner-nation capacity-building efforts in Iraq and Syria during this time because longer-term capacity-building efforts were not supported under the Counter-Islamic State of Iraq and Syria (ISIS) Train and Equip Fund (discussions with U.S. defense officials, March 2, 2021).

[80] Discussions with U.S. defense officials, March 2, 2021, and March 9, 2021.

AFRICOM GHE Activities Focus on Infectious Disease Preparedness and Medical Support Capabilities

GHE in AFRICOM has historically focused primarily on infectious disease preparedness and response. GHE activities in AFRICOM have been conducted under the DoD HIV/AIDS Prevention Program and through such initiatives as the African Partnership Outbreak Response Alliance.[81] AFRICOM has been particularly active in the Africa Malaria Task Force, working with countries in East and West Africa to combat malaria through rapid response team training and tabletop exercises.[82] In March 2019, AFRICOM and the Ugandan Ministries of Defense and Health cohosted the Africa Malaria Task Force, bringing experts from 18 African partner countries, nongovernmental organizations, and other nonprofit organizations together to share best practices and lessons learned for malaria control.[83]

Medical personnel in AFRICOM also provide combat casualty care and evacuation training to partner militaries as part of broader counterterrorism and peacekeeping operations missions. Special operations forces and the air component (USAFE-AFAFRICA) are involved in these training efforts.[84] Another major effort involves the African Peacekeeping Rapid Response Partnership (APRRP) program, which provides medical equipment and training for six countries.[85] AFRICOM's naval component, U.S. Naval Forces Europe-Africa, has conducted combat casualty care training and has provided four African partner countries with training and equipment to efficiently and effectively set up, take down, and operate a United Nations–standard Level 2 hospital through APRRP.[86] The USUHS's Center for Global Health Engagement contributed to the effort by providing education and training activities and exercises to ensure that African partner countries have the capacity to rapidly deploy and sustain these mobile field hospitals.[87] Although these hospitals are intended to support peacekeeping missions,

---

[81] The African Partnership Outbreak Response Alliance is an African-led, AFRICOM-facilitated series of key leader engagements that focus on building health security capacities among partner nations while promoting effective military-civilian partnerships (Global Health Security Agenda, *Strengthening Health Security Across the Globe: Progress and Impact of U.S. Government Investments in the Global Health Security Agenda*, October 2021; and discussion with AFRICOM GHE personnel, November 24, 2020).

[82] Discussions with U.S. defense officials, January 14, 2021.

[83] Grady Jones, "AFRICOM Africa Malaria Taskforce Key Leader Event–2019 Comes to a Close," U.S. Africa Command, April 15, 2019.

[84] Tactical Combat Casualty Care and CASEVAC training were started by U.S. special operations forces, then continued by members of the 818th Mobility Support Advisory Squadron (AFRICOM, 2019; and discussions with DoD officials, January 26, 2021).

[85] APRRP is most active in Uganda, Rwanda, Senegal, and Ghana. APRRP provided $6.5 million to equip two mobile hospitals each in Senegal and Ghana and approximately $2 million each to be used for training (AFRICOM, "AFRICOM's Partnership Endures During COVID-19," April 14, 2020).

[86] Discussions with DoD personnel, November 24, 2020.

[87] Uniformed Services University Center for Global Health Engagement, "Programs and Operational Support," webpage, undated.

Ghana, Senegal, and Uganda each deployed their mobile hospitals to provide needed medical capabilities in the region in response to the COVID-19 pandemic.[88]

AFRICOM's GHE activities have primarily focused on pandemic response and providing humanitarian assistance. However, by developing field hospitals and providing tactical casualty care and CASEVAC training, AFRICOM has also contributed to increasing the capacity of African nations to provide expeditionary medical care.[89] These efforts decrease the need for external assistance and support the combatant command's broader lines of effort related to improving regional stability.[90]

SOUTHCOM Activities Focus on Public Health Engagement and Medical Readiness Training and Exercises

In SOUTHCOM, GHE activities have focused on (1) building the capabilities of partners to provide effective medical care for local populations and (2) providing opportunities for training U.S. forces.[91] Our discussions with GHE personnel assigned to the region also revealed that there has been a push since 2017 to organize conferences on infectious disease monitoring and response; the Global Health Security of the Americas Conference, held in Panama in March 2019, is a recent example.[92] Health efforts focused on vaccine distribution during the COVID-19 pandemic, but components in SOUTHCOM have continued to work with partner militaries to improve their biosurveillance capabilities more broadly and with the Pan American Health Organization to improve field hospitals and emergency medical response capabilities throughout the region.[93]

Disaster response exercises often have a medical component, providing an opportunity to deliver training to partner militaries in this area.[94] Many of these exercises are conducted by Joint Task Force-Bravo, which engages with partner countries when deployed to the region for crisis response missions.[95] Special forces civil affairs teams also engage in small-scale activities aimed at improving local medical capabilities and strengthening civil networks, while conventional service components have been working with regional leaders in countries such as Colombia to

---

[88] Discussions with DoD personnel, November 24, 2020.

[89] Discussions with DoD personnel, November 24, 2020; and AFRICOM, 2019.

[90] AFRICOM, 2019.

[91] Discussions with DoD officials, March 10, 2021.

[92] Discussions with DoD officials, March 10, 2021.

[93] Discussions with DoD officials, March 4, 2021.

[94] Discussions with DoD officials March 10, 2021.

[95] Joint Task Force-Bravo has a designated medical element that conducts GHE activities (SOUTHCOM, "U.S. Military Wraps Up Disaster Relief Exercise in Belize," January 18, 2022).

make them capability exporters in the areas of health care system development and patient movement and evacuation.[96]

A major focus of the air component in SOUTHCOM is on Medical Readiness Training Exercises (MEDRETEs). MEDRETEs are designed to provide humanitarian assistance and free medical care to the people of the host nation while helping improve the skills of U.S. military medical forces and the military medical professionals of the host nation. These exercises are particularly helpful in aiding in U.S. medical readiness by providing surgical units with the opportunity to train in a realistic, austere environment.[97] Similarly, annual exercises such as RESOLUTE SENTINEL contribute to medical readiness by engaging with partner militaries in training for disaster response and increasing interoperability.[98] DoD officials noted that partner countries regularly request engagements to build their capabilities related to aeromedical evacuation, people movement, and transportation.[99]

A study of GHE activities from 2012 to 2017 in three SOUTHCOM countries—El Salvador, Guatemala, and Honduras—found that 64 percent of the 414 activities conducted by the GCC and components were focused on providing direct care, and the most common of the reported objectives for these activities was U.S. operational readiness, as opposed to security cooperation or health outcome objectives.[100] The emphasis on finding opportunities for increasing U.S. medical readiness by providing health care through MEDRETEs and embedded medical teams was also highlighted by U.S. defense officials as a primary goal of GHE in SOUTHCOM.[101]

Table 2.1 summarizes the main GHE priorities and activities across the five GCCs included in our study.

---

[96] Discussions with DoD officials, February 25, 2021, and March 10, 2021.

[97] Discussions with U.S. defense officials, March 10, 2021, and March 25, 2022; and 12th Air Force, "Medical Readiness Training Exercises (MEDRETEs)," webpage, undated.

[98] Discussions with U.S. defense officials, March 25, 2021.

[99] Discussions with DoD officials, March 10, 2021.

[100] Casey Perez, Diana Aguirre, Brian Neese, Joshua Vess, and Edwin K. Burkett, "Evaluating Team Characteristics for Health Engagements in Three Countries in Central America: 2012–2017," *Military Medicine*, July 6, 2021.

[101] Discussions with DoD officials, March 4, 2021.

Table 2.1. Summary of GHE Programs and Activities Across the GCCs

GCC	Programs and Activities	
INDOPACOM	• Enhancing public health and support for humanitarian disasters • Providing access for potential contingencies • Increasing regional military medical capabilities	• Public health outreach • Disease surveillance and trauma care exchanges • MEDEVAC and CASEVAC exercises
EUCOM	• Expanding expeditionary medical capacity • Increasing NATO interoperability	• Role 1 and Role 2 capability expert exchanges[a] • Medical logistics exercises
CENTCOM	• Improving regional trauma care for current operations	• Trauma care facility support • Personnel exchanges and embeds • MEDEVAC exercises
AFRICOM	• Increasing partner capacity to respond to infectious diseases • Developing medical support capabilities for counterterrorism and peacekeeping	• Preventive medicine education and training • Partner CASEVAC and trauma care training
SOUTHCOM	• Building regional medical response capabilities • Increasing public health capacity and opportunities for U.S. medical training	• Public health outreach • MEDRETEs

SOURCES: Discussions with DoD officials and GCC briefings.

[a] Role 1 capability is known as *first responder care* and involves providing immediate life-saving measures. Role 2 capability includes more-advanced trauma management and emergency medical treatment and provides a greater capability to resuscitate patients. Full definitions for Role 1 and Role 2 capabilities can be found in Joint Publication 4-02, *Joint Health Services*, Joint Chiefs of Staff, Incorporating Change 1, September 28, 2018.

GCC GHE Activities Increasingly Focus on Force Health Protection and Medical Readiness

Our research and discussions with GHE personnel across the combatant commands indicate that although GCC GHE activities reflect different regional priorities, they share a common focus on force health protection and medical readiness. GHE stakeholders in each theater recognized a growing need to work with allies and partners to increase their medical capacity and improve their degree of interoperability with the United States, either to ensure the health and safety of U.S. and allied forces or to develop sufficient medical support for a future contingency.

In INDOPACOM, GHE activities related to disease surveillance and preventive medicine have become more closely linked to force protection objectives since the outbreak of the COVID-19 pandemic. At the same time, increased demand for engagements and training exercises aimed at improving partner nations' trauma care and MEDEVAC capabilities has been driven by a need to improve medical readiness across the region in the event of a contingency.

In EUCOM, GHE activities aimed at developing NATO-standard Role 1 and Role 2 capabilities in Eastern Europe are directly related to U.S. and allied medical readiness objectives. Interest in expanding GHE activities to engage in additional medical logistics exercises and develop greater interoperability among Western European countries and the United States appears to reflect evolving concerns about the need for medical support in a potential or expanding conflict in Europe. Similarly, in CENTCOM, GHE activities that focus on developing trauma care facilities and MEDEVAC capabilities in the Middle East relate to an ongoing desire to improve medical readiness in the Middle East and the Persian Gulf to ensure seamless tactical support during contingency operations.

In AFRICOM and SOUTHCOM, GHE has historically been viewed as supporting soft power objectives; however, CASEVAC and trauma care training for peacekeeping operations and the development of United Nations–standard expeditionary medical facilities in African countries are also related to medical readiness and force protection objectives. ADM Craig S. Faller, the former head of SOUTHCOM, described the medical outreach efforts by USNS Comfort as a means of "strengthening collective medical readiness and interoperability" across Latin America and the Caribbean.[102] Moreover, DoD interest in expanding MEDRETEs in South America to provide additional training opportunities for U.S. medical personnel is further evidence that GHE is seen as a means to increase U.S. readiness worldwide.

In summary, we found that although medical planners in each GCC and component have undertaken different approaches to tying GHE to broader strategic objectives and have pursued various GHE activities according to the operational requirements within their theater, they expressed a common interest in investing more in developing partner medical capabilities and capacity to ensure medical readiness and force protection. In the next chapter, we discuss the various sources of funding that medical planners use to support GHE activities in each of the GCCs and the challenges they have in meeting their respective objectives.

---

[102] Craig S. Faller, "A Collective Presence in the Western Hemisphere Reduces Threats to the US and Its Allies," *Defense News*, September 5, 2019.

Chapter 3. Challenges in Meeting GHE Priorities with Current Funding

Obtaining funding for GHE activities is a persistent challenge. Like all security cooperation planners, GHE stakeholders face obstacles in navigating the patchwork of authorities, organizations, and procedures required to acquire the necessary personnel and resources to conduct activities with allies and partners.[103] What makes GHE planning particularly challenging is the lack of a dedicated source of funding for health-related activities and the difficulty in obtaining the consistent, multiyear support necessary to develop partner medical capacity and interoperable capabilities.

GHE planners must therefore rely on short-term funding sources that vary in applicability and availability by region and type of activity. As we note in Chapter 1, GHE has expanded so widely over the past two decades that many members of the DoD community lack a clear understanding of the purpose of global health activities. Moreover, GHE is not viewed as way to achieve operational objectives and is not prioritized in security cooperation planning.

In this chapter, we describe the primary, often regionally specific, sources of funding that each of the GCCs has relied on to support GHE activities. We depict the major challenges GHE stakeholders have faced in addressing their priorities with limited and inconsistent sources of support, then address the implications of the lack of multiyear funding.

GCCs Rely on Distinct Funding Streams to Implement GHE Activities

Just as GHE activities vary across GCCs, we found that each command relies on distinct funding streams. Components use both Title 10 and Title 22 funding sources that are authorized by DoD and the Department of State, respectively, to support their activities, but the mix of available sources is different in each geographic region.[104] Each type of funding has its own

---

[103] The complexity of U.S. security cooperation funding has been the subject of numerous studies, including Beth Grill, Michael J. McNerney, Jeremy Boback, Renanah Miles, Cynthia C. Clapp-Wincek, and David E. Thaler, *Follow the Money: Promoting Greater Transparency in Department of Defense Security Cooperation Reporting*, RAND Corporation, RR-2039-OSD, 2017; and David E. Thaler, Michael J. McNerney, Beth Grill, Jefferson P. Marquis, and Amanda Kadlec, *From Patchwork to Framework: A Review of Title 10 Authorities for Security Cooperation*, RAND Corporation, RR-1438-OSD, 2016.

[104] Title 22 funds are appropriated to the U.S. Department of State and then transferred to DoD to manage and execute security assistance programs. These funds are authorized by Congress and appropriated on a by-country and by-program basis. Title 22 funds include Foreign Military Sales (FMS) programs. Title 10 funds are appropriated directly to DoD and intended for operations and maintenance of the U.S. military. They are often used to fund international participation in U.S. joint exercises, military personnel exchanges, or military-to-military contacts to build and strengthen relationships between partner military and U.S forces. GHE activities conducted by the State

restrictions and limitations, yet a common problem across all funding sources is a lack of consistent support for building partner capacity and interoperability with U.S. forces.

Asia Pacific Regional Initiative Is a Primary Source of GHE Funding in INDOPACOM

DoD officials indicated that the primary source of funding for GHE activities in the INDOPACOM region was provided through the Asia Pacific Regional Initiative (APRI), a Title 10 authority designated by Congress to support theater security cooperation activities in the Pacific, such as humanitarian assistance and payment of incremental and personnel costs of training and exercising with foreign security forces.[105] In 2020, APRI funding totaled $14 million for all combatant command activities.[106] A small portion of those funds was used to support individual GHE military-to-military engagements, such as subject-matter expert exchanges on issues of disease surveillance and trauma care, and to support public health outreach efforts in Southeast Asia and Oceania. APRI funding is provided to the INDOPACOM combatant commander on an annual basis. It cannot be used to support long-term activities.

INDOPACOM also receives some support for GHE outreach activities to civilian organizations through Overseas Humanitarian, Disaster, and Civic Aid (OHDACA), a single appropriation that includes several Title 10 authorities, including an authority dedicated specifically to humanitarian assistance.[107] OHDACA-funded activities are limited to those short-term activities that provide direct benefits to civilian populations rather than partner militaries. Although DSCA manages OHDACA funds, the combatant command determines which proposals are submitted for funding. A third source of funding for GHE activities in INDOPACOM comes from service Operation and Maintenance (O&M) funds, which are allocated by the services. These funds cover the costs of Army key leader engagements, Air Force participation in PACIFIC ANGEL exercises, and the Navy's involvement in the Pacific Partnership program.

GHE stakeholders in the service components indicated that other types of funding can be used to support individual medical-related activities, such as the IMET program, which supports military training for foreign military personnel at U.S. military schools and programs, and HCA funds, which support the local population in conjunction with U.S. exercises. In some cases, HCA contributes to a portion of a mission. As one stakeholder noted, for Pacific Partnership missions, medical planners rely on a combination of APRI, service O&M, and HCA funding.

Partnership Program may also be supported through Title 32 authorities, which support the U.S. National Guard (Terrence K. Kelly, Jefferson P. Marquis, Cathryn Quantic Thurston, Jennifer D. P. Moroney, and Charlotte Lynch, *Security Cooperation Organizations in the Country Team: Options for Success*, RAND Corporation, TR-734-A, 2010).

[105] Public Law 115-31, Consolidated Appropriations Act, 2017, May 5, 2017.

[106] Defense Security Cooperation University, *Security Cooperation Programs Handbook for Fiscal Year 2020*, 2020, p. 123.

[107] U.S. Code, Title 10, Section 2561, Humanitarian Assistance.

(Service O&M provides support for personnel costs and ship costs, while HCA covers the costs of medical supplies used on shore.[108]) Each of these funds are for a single year only.

It is also important to note that countries in the region receive support for GHE-related activities through other funding sources beyond Title 10 or Title 22 security cooperation programs, such as the Biological Threat Reduction Program (BTRP), which is a part of the Title 50 Cooperative Threat Reduction program that supports biosurveillance training and facilities. BTRP is overseen by DTRA, which determines funding allocations. DTRA can allocate funds over a three-year time frame. However, although BTRP is conducted alongside GCC activities, it is not under the purview or direction of the GCC and is not part of the security cooperation planning process.

Medical planners in INDPACOM noted that there were significant restrictions on how each funding source could be applied to GHE. APRI funds could only be used for military-to-military contacts—not for equipping, training, or infrastructure—and could only provide support for U.S. service personnel to conduct activities in a single fiscal year. O&M funds used for other military-to-military visits and exercises are also limited and cannot be used for BPC. On the other hand, OHDACA funds can only be used to provide direct support to civilians; these funds are prohibited from supporting partner-nation military forces. Other funding sources, such as BTRP, are limited in scope and are not within INDOPACOM's ability to influence or control. Moreover, none of the funding mechanisms on which the GCC relies for GHE is designated for medical purposes; therefore, GHE activities are often not prioritized for funding by the combatant command, the services, or DoD agencies. Thus, the only sources of funding have been single-year allocations that support on-time events. Moreover, the funding for these events has been limited, often falling below the "cut line" of the GCCs, as will be discussed in more detail in the next chapter.

European Deterrence Initiative Is a Primary Source of GHE Funding in EUCOM

In the European theater, the primary source of funding is the European Deterrence Initiative (EDI). EDI is a congressionally authorized initiative designed to "enhance the U.S. deterrence posture, increase the readiness and responsiveness of U.S. forces in Europe, support the collective defense and security of NATO allies, and bolster the security and capacity of U.S. allies and partners."[109] The EUCOM combatant commander can influence how EDI funds are allocated within these four bins. EDI funds have been used to support as much as 95 percent of EUCOM's GHE activities, according to one DoD official.[110] However, GHE stakeholders

---

[108] Discussions with U.S. defense officials, April 29, 2021.

[109] EDI was established by the Obama administration and authorized by Congress in 2014 under the initial title of the European Reassurance Initiative. It was renamed EDI in 2018 (Paul Belkin and Hibbah Kaileh, "The European Deterrence Initiative: A Budgetary Overview," Congressional Research Service, IF10946, July 1, 2021, p. 1).

[110] Discussions with DoD officials, November 6, 2020, and March 24, 2021.

indicated that EDI funds have been limited to supporting subject-matter expert exchanges and certification of Role 1 and Role 2 facilities, as nearly all have been supported by funds designated for "USEUCOM Engagements."[111] These military-to-military engagement funds can only be used to cover personnel costs for meetings or information exchange and cannot be used for the purposes of capacity-building.[112] Although other EDI funds have been designated to support U.S. Army prepositioned medical assets and U.S. Air Force Health Service Support equipment in Europe, no EDI funds have been used to develop partner-nation capacity in any country aside from Ukraine. Thus, they have not been used to provide direct infrastructure support for the building of Role 1 or Role 2 facilities for partner nations.[113] Until fiscal year 2022, EDI was funded through DoD's Overseas Contingency Operations (OCO) funds, rather than the base budget. Unlike DoD's Future Years Defense Program, which includes projected funding over five years, OCO funding was typically planned for one year at a time.

In addition to EDI, medical planners indicated that they use Traditional Combatant Command Activities (TCA) funds to support GHE activities. TCA can be allocated by a GCC commander for military-to-military contacts and comparable activities. It has been used to support subject-matter expert exchanges and visits to medical facilities. In addition, service O&M funds provide support to regional exercises in the European theater that include a medical component. O&M funds supported MEDEVAC training in Poland that preceded the ALLIED SPIRIT readiness exercise with NATO countries, for example.[114]

Other small amounts of funding for medical-related activities are supported by institutional capacity-building funds. Prior to 2021, the Wales Initiative Fund (WIF) supported institutional capacity-building efforts in countries that participate in the NATO Partnership for Peace program.[115] WIF was used to support exchanges, exercises, and workshops supporting NATO interoperability, which could include medical capacity-building. It also supported a Ministry of

---

[111] Discussion with DoD official, March 24, 2021.

[112] Military-to-military engagements funds are limited to covering the costs of National Guard Bureau personnel pay and allowances and TCA (Office of the Under Secretary of Defense [Comptroller], *European Deterrence Initiative: Department of Defense Budget Fiscal Year [FY] 2023*, April 2022, p. 18).

[113] EDI designates funding for combat medical support for the U.S. Army and for the Air Force Health Services operating in Europe under the Enhanced Prepositioning Line of Effort. The only funding for medical support under the Building Partner Capacity Line of Effort is designated for Ukraine as part of the Ukraine Security Assistance effort. This funding provides training and equipment for military medical treatment. See Office of the Under Secretary of Defense (Comptroller), *European Deterrence Initiative: Department of Defense Budget Fiscal Year (FY) 2020*, March 2019; and Office of the Under Secretary of Defense (Comptroller), *European Deterrence Initiative: Department of Defense Budget Fiscal Year (FY) 2021*, February 2020b.

[114] Mniedlo, 2020.

[115] WIF, previously known as the Warsaw Initiative Fund, supported defense reform efforts and institutional capacity-building in 16 Eastern European and Central Asian countries that participate in the Partnership for Peace program. Since 2021, WIF and Partnership for Peace activities have been supported by International Security Cooperation Programs Account funds and regional centers.

Defense Advisors program in Ukraine.[116] These activities previously supported by WIF are now supported by the Security Cooperation Programs Account and regional centers, which fund defense institution-building, military-to-military contacts, payment of expenses to attend bilateral or regional conferences, and payment of training and exercise expenses to foreign partners.[117]

GHE stakeholders indicated that although EUCOM uses OHDACA funding less frequently when compared with other GCCs, OHDACA funds have been tapped to provide support to several countries to assist in COVID-19 pandemic relief efforts.[118] Moreover, stakeholders also noted that DTRA funding has supported biosurveillance and testing efforts through DoD's support for biological surveillance networks.[119]

Nevertheless, DoD officials from EUCOM noted that each of these funding mechanisms for GHE activities has limitations. TCA funding can only support military-to-military contacts, such as knowledge exchanges and familiarization visits. Similar to APRI in INDOPACOM, TCA funds cannot be used to support equipping, training, infrastructure, or other long-term engagements. EDI support has been limited to supporting subject-matter expert exchanges and familiarization visits by U.S. personnel (aside from Ukraine).[120] Moreover, although O&M funding can be used for medical activities in the context of military exercises, developing interoperable military medical support is often not a priority, and such funding only allows for intermittent engagement with Western Europe partners in the EUCOM theater. As with INDOPACOM, funding has only been provided to support individual engagements in a single fiscal year.

CENTCOM Relies on Partner-Funded Foreign Military Sales to Support GHE Activities

CENTCOM does not have a regional funding source that is similar to APRI or EDI. As a result, CENTCOM components rely primarily on limited TCA funds allocated by the combatant

---

[116] EUCOM Global Health Engagement Working Group, briefing, August 12, 2020, Not available to the general public.

[117] Defense Security Cooperation University, *Security Cooperation Programs Handbook for Fiscal Year 2021*, 2021, p. 167; and Office of the Under Secretary of Defense (Comptroller), "Fiscal Year 2022 President's Budget: Defense Security Cooperation Agency," May 2021.

[118] EUCOM, "FY 2020 European Deterrence Initiative (EDI) Fact Sheet," undated.

[119] EUCOM Global Health Engagement Working Group, 2020; and David Vergun, "DOD Supports Partner Nations with COVID-19 Mitigation Assistance," U.S. Department of Defense, June 1, 2020.

[120] Although some BPC efforts are permitted to be funded under EDI, GHE stakeholders noted that EDI had not been authorized for anything beyond subject-matter expert exchanges and familiarization visits. Additionally, DoD officials indicated that EDI was unlikely to be authorized for additional BPC activities that might include GHE. Moreover, they noted that GHE funding was expected to decline significantly in the FY 2022 budget. However, since the February 2022 Russian invasion of Ukraine, EDI funding has only declined slightly, from $4.5 billion in FY 2021 to $3.8 billion in FY 2023. DoD's EDI funding request for FY 2023 totals $4.2 billion (conference call with GHE stakeholders, September 7, 2021; and Office of the Under Secretary of Defense (Comptroller) and Chief Financial Officer, *Defense Budget Overview: United States Department of Defense Fiscal Year 2023 Budget Request*, April 2022, pp. 3–4).

commander to support GHE activities. TCA funds support one-time events, such as information and subject-matter expert exchanges.[121] The only other major source of funding is through institutional capacity-building programs, such as WIF, which provides support for Central Asian countries that are eligible to receive NATO Partnership for Peace support as former Soviet states. WIF funds (which are now incorporated into other funding programs for institutional capacity-building) have been used to support information and subject-matter expert exchanges related to health.

During our discussions, medical planners in AFCENT and other service components said that they have also used O&M funding to practice operating with partner nations' medical personnel during exercises, although the amount of service O&M funding devoted to medical training is limited, and there have been few other ways to support training on combat casualty management and MEDEVAC outside Afghanistan.[122]

Unlike in the other GCCs, U.S. partners in CENTCOM have invested a significant amount of their own funds toward developing interoperable medical capabilities through the Foreign Military Sales (FMS) program. As noted above, the UAE has invested $44 million in an FMS case to develop a joint, multinational Trauma, Burn, and Rehabilitative Medicine program.[123] This investment provides the UAE with advising, training, mentoring, and technical support, as well as the opportunity to work closely with U.S. medical personnel as they exercise their trauma care skills.[124] In addition to FMS, CENTCOM GHE activities are funded through other security assistance programs managed by the State Department, such as IMET and the Global Peace Operations Initiative (GPOI), which is one of several peacekeeping operations funds intended to enhance international capacity to conduct United Nations and regional peace support operations by building partner country capabilities to train and sustain peacekeeping proficiencies.[125] IMET and GPOI funds support education and training engagements conducted in Kazakhstan, for example.[126] However, these Title 22 programs are planned and funded through different processes than other GCC Title 10 programs.[127]

Overall, there has been relatively less funding available for conducting trauma care and MEDEVAC training in the CENTCOM theater than in INDOPACOM or EUCOM. Aside from

---

[121] TCA funds are primarily used to support engagements in the Levant and Arabian Peninsula (discussion with U.S. defense officials, March 11, 2021).

[122] Although the status of the Afghan Security Forces Fund was unknown at the time of this writing, training and advising activities were no longer occurring in Afghanistan.

[123] Discussion with U.S. defense officials, March 2, 2021; and Richard Bumgardner, "Medical Ties Bind Forces in Partnership," *Army Magazine*, Vol. 70, No. 8, August 2020.

[124] Discussion with U.S. defense officials, March 2, 2021; and Licina and Taylor, 2022.

[125] Discussion with U.S. defense officials, March 2, 2021.

[126] Discussion with U.S. defense officials, March 9, 2021.

[127] Discussion with U.S. defense officials, March 9, 2021.

partner-funded FMS activities, DoD officials noted that, in most cases, they only have limited, short-term funding available to conduct military-to-military exchanges.[128] Medical planners also indicated that they have had difficulty integrating FMS-funded activities into other GHE engagements, which are supported through different processes.

AFRICOM Relies Primarily on Department of State Title 22 Funding to Support GHE Activities

In the AFRICOM theater, there are no designated regional security cooperation funds, and less TCA support is available for military-to-military engagements in comparison with other regions. Title 10 funding for partnership capacity-building support is also limited. Medical personnel in AFRICOM and across the service components rely primarily on a mix of U.S.-funded Title 22 security assistance programs to support their engagement with partner nations. These Title 22 programs are often tied to broader public health or stability efforts. One of the region's major sources of GHE funding is the President's Emergency Plan for AIDS Relief (PEPFAR), which supports the DoD HIV/AIDS Prevention Program.[129] The DoD HIV/AIDS Prevention Program provides funding to support U.S. military personnel working with partner military medical organizations in several countries; however, these funds can only be used to address HIV/AIDS and related complications.[130]

Other major sources of funding in AFRICOM include the Partnership for Regional East Africa Counterterrorism (PREACT), the Trans-Sahara Counterterrorism Partnership (TSCTP), and the APRRP. These funds support U.S. efforts to train and equip African military forces in designated countries to conduct counterterrorism and peacekeeping missions. Although these funds are not designated specifically for medical care, some of these engagements include the provision of training and equipment for tactical combat care and evacuation.[131] Together, these three programs support most military-to-military capacity-building efforts with African partner nations.

Like other GCCs, AFRICOM relies on O&M funding to support information exchanges and education efforts related to infectious disease containment; the African Partnership Outbreak Response Alliance is an example of such efforts. Service components also rely on their own O&M funds to support outreach efforts, such as African Partnership Flight and African Partnership Station, and to conduct exercises and port visits, some of which may include a medical component. DoD officials noted that some training and equipping for medical capabilities may be included in activities funded through Foreign Military Financing or Section

---

[128] Discussions with U.S. defense officials, March 9, 2021.

[129] DoD serves as the executive agent for the administration of efforts to support AIDS prevention, care, and treatment for foreign militaries under this State Department–managed Title 22 program.

[130] Discussions with U.S. defense official, April 29, 2021.

[131] AFRICOM, 2019.

333 building partnership capacity-building cases but that such funding was rarely used for GHE activities in the AFRICOM theater.

Section 333 of Title 10 provides DoD with the authority to build the capacity of partner nations—which includes equipment and training—to enable them to conduct one or more of the following activities: counterterrorism operations, counter–weapons of mass destruction, counter–illicit drug trafficking operations, counter–transnational crime, maritime and border security operations, military intelligence operations, air domain awareness, cyberspace or defensive cyberspace operations, and international coalition operations.[132] This authority, previously known as the Section 1206 Train and Equip Program, was focused on counterterrorism when it was established in 2006 but has expanded over time. According to one defense official, Congress is considering expanding the authority to include capacity-building efforts to enable humanitarian operations.[133]

Funding for Section 333 programs is provided through a competitive process, with proposals submitted though the GCC to the Office of the Secretary of Defense and the Joint Staff for approval.[134] Once funding is awarded, it may be distributed over two fiscal years. According to one defense official, Section 333 funding may have been used to support medical efforts tied to maritime defense and borders security; however, such use of these Section 333 funds has been very rare.[135]

In most cases, O&M funds have been limited to single-year allocations that support on-time events. As a result, AFRICOM has been unable to support planned multiyear medical engagements and has achieved only a fraction of its objectives.[136] Title 22–funded activities have allowed for training and equipping, although health typically has not been a key focus of such activities and often is not prioritized. Overall, this lack of consistent funding limits continuity and forces AFRICOM GHE personnel to rebuild their portfolios each year.[137]

Although OHDACA was not mentioned by stakeholders as a major source of GHE funding during our discussions, OHDACA support was mentioned as part of the COVID-19 pandemic response effort. According to a DoD Inspector General report, AFRICOM received as much as $21 million in humanitarian assistance funding from March 2020 to June 2021 to respond to the pandemic. This funding was used to conduct 27 health projects to assist civilians in partner

---

[132] U.S. Code, Title 10, Section 333, Foreign Security Forces: Authority to Build Capacity.

[133] Discussion with U.S. defense officials, September 7, 2020.

[134] Defense Security Cooperation Agency, "Section 333 Authority to Build Capacity," webpage, undated-c.

[135] Discussion with U.S. defense officials, September 7, 2020.

[136] Discussions with DoD officials, November 24, 2020.

[137] Discussions with DoD officials, November 24, 2020.

nations across the AFRICOM area of responsibility. COVID-19 pandemic assistance included support for mobile field hospitals, isolation clinics, medical equipment, and medical supplies.[138]

SOUTHCOM Relies Primarily on OHDACA Funds

SOUTHCOM, like AFRICOM, has limited sources of funding available for GHE. Most medical engagements in this theater are funded through OHDACA funds, which can be used to conduct GHE missions dedicated to supporting humanitarian assistance. The only other source of GHE support is provided by SOUTHCOM and service O&M funds. These O&M funds support MEDRETEs that aim to enhance partners' medical care capabilities while improving the readiness of U.S. partner-nation military medical forces.[139] U.S. Navy O&M funds also support the operations of USNS Comfort, which supports GHE engagements through the Continuing Promise and Enduring Promise initiatives.[140] Additionally, SOUTHCOM uses exercise support and HCA funding to enable the participation of U.S. forces in development activities within the context of military exercises, training, or operations. However, these funds do not constitute a significant source of GHE support. Several officials noted that the service components have sought to use Section 333 train and equip authorities to support health-related capacity-building initiatives with partner militaries but, to date, have not been successful in having their proposals funded.[141]

DoD officials pointed out that, unlike other regions, SOUTHCOM has not been designated to receive support from the Cooperative Threat Reduction program; therefore, the GCC does not receive any biosurveillance funds through DTRA's BTRP.[142] Stakeholders in the region indicated that this has been a limiting factor in DoD's ability to support broader global health activities.[143] Table 3.1 summarizes the major differences in GHE priorities, activities, and sources of funding across the GCCs.

---

[138] U.S. Department of Defense Office of Inspector General, *Audit of U.S. Africa Command's Execution of Coronavirus Aid, Relief, and Economic Security Act Funding*, March 31, 2022, p. 4.

[139] 12th Air Force, undated.

[140] The Continuing Promise and Enduring Promise initiatives also receive support from SOUTHCOM OHDACA funds.

[141] Discussions with U.S. defense officials, March 4, 2021.

[142] Discussions with U.S. defense officials, March 4, 2021.

[143] Discussions with U.S. defense officials, March 4, 2021.

Table 3.1. GHE Priorities, Activities, and Sources of Funding Across the GCCs

GCC	GHE Priorities	Primary Activities	Primary Funding Sources
INDOPACOM	• Enhancing public health and support for humanitarian disasters • Providing access for potential contingencies • Increasing regional military medical capabilities	• Public health outreach • Disease surveillance and trauma care exchanges • MEDEVAC and CASEVAC exercises	• APRI • OHDACA • Service O&M funding
EUCOM	• Expanding expeditionary medical capacity • Increasing NATO interoperability	• Role 1 and Role 2 capability expert exchanges • Medical logistics exercises	• EDI • TCA
CENTCOM	• Improving regional trauma care for current operations	• Trauma care facility support • Personnel exchanges and embeds • MEDEVAC exercises	• FMS • TCA
AFRICOM	• Increasing partner capacity to respond to infectious diseases • Developing medical support capabilities for counterterrorism and peacekeeping	• Preventive medicine education and training • Partner CASEVAC and trauma care training	• PEPFAR • PREACT • TSCTP • APRRP
SOUTHCOM	• Building regional medical response capabilities • Increasing public health capacity and opportunities for U.S. medical training	• Public health outreach • MEDRETEs	• OHDACA • O&M funding

SOURCE: Features information from stakeholder discussions and GCC briefings.

Notably, DoD officials did not refer to the Defense Health Program (DHP) as a source of funding for GHE activities. DHP is a sub-account under the O&M account that funds military health system functions for U.S. forces. The primary purpose of the program is to deliver patient care through military treatment facilities or health care providers participating in TRICARE, the DoD-administered health insurance–like program. DHP also supports certain medical readiness activities and expeditionary medical capabilities; education and training programs; research, development, test, and evaluation; management and headquarters activities; facilities sustainment; procurement; and civilian and contract personnel.[144] DHP supports professional military education programs that include foreign partners through the USUHS and other activities that involve partner nations, but it is not a security cooperation fund.

DHP funds also support research activities supported through a grant mechanism by which DoD funds, such as Army Medical Research Acquisition Activity funds, are provided to the

---

[144] Bryce H. P. Mendez, "FY2022 Budget Request for the Military Health System," Congressional Research Service, IF11856, June 15, 2021; and U.S. Code, Title 10, Section 1100, Defense Health Program Account.

Henry M. Jackson Foundation and then distributed over multiple years to a miliary medical research institution.[145] The Jackson Foundation is a nonprofit organization established by Congress in 1983 to support research at the USUHS and other military medical entities.[146] This type of grant mechanism is rare. Although DTRA also provides some grants through organizations for the purposes of research and development, this funding may not be applicable to areas of GHE beyond dedicated research programs. Funding for security cooperation engagements with partner nations must follow designated timelines for the obligation and expenditure of funds. As noted in Appendix A, most Title 10–funded programs, which are supported with O&M funds, must be expended within one year.

In this chapter, we described the various funding mechanisms that GCCs use to conduct GHE activities. GHE stakeholders clearly noted that each funding source presents challenges to conducting consistent engagement with partner nations. Interestingly, however, none of the officials we spoke with referred specifically to a need to establish a dedicated funding source for GHE or a GHE program of record. Instead, most focused on the need to prioritize GHE activities for funding across the GCCs and to more explicitly link GHE to theater operational priorities or depict GHE within an ends-ways-means framework. Many officials stressed the importance of being able to draw on multiyear funding sources in order to build medical capacity and interoperable medical capabilities. Yet they indicated that GHE stakeholders often have difficulty communicating to senior leadership why GHE engagements are necessary, how they link to a GCC commander's theater plans, and why the military's medical force is well-positioned to advance the objectives. In the next chapter, we discuss these findings in more depth and consider the types of funding options that could be pursued to better support GHE activities linked to GCC objectives.

---

[145] Cause IQ, "Henry M Jackson Foundation for the Advancement of Military Medicine," webpage, undated.

[146] Kellie Moss and Josh Michaud, *The U.S. Department of Defense and Global Health: Infectious Disease Efforts*, Kaiser Family Foundation, October 2013.

Chapter 4. Summary and Recommendations

Nearly all the GHE stakeholders we had discussions with indicated that inconsistent funding limited the ability of GCCs to build long-term medical capacity and capabilities. Moreover, they noted that a lack of prioritization of GHE has made it difficult for GHE proposals to compete against other security cooperation activities that are more explicitly tied to operational objectives. Many officials expressed a strong need for improved approaches to funding GHE across the GCCs, and some provided ideas for what an ideal source of GHE funding might look like. In this chapter, we discuss these findings in more detail, then outline our recommendations for improving support to GHE.

Findings

Inconsistent, Short-Term Funding Limits GCCs' Ability to Build Medical Capacity and Capabilities

Our conversations with DoD personnel indicated that a lack of reliable and consistent funding is a significant challenge in planning and conducting GHE activities. Although each of the GCCs relies on different sources of funds to support health engagements, nearly all available funding sources are limited to supporting one-time events or activities that occur in a single fiscal year. Moreover, much of this funding is restricted to supporting military-to-military visits and subject-matter expert exchanges. (According to one DoD official with a global perspective, 60–70 percent of all GHE activities are supported by military-to-military funding.[147]) Planners cannot rely on funding to be available from year to year or to provide consistent training engagements over time. This makes it difficult for GCCs and components to plan and execute GHE activities aimed at building partner medical capacity and developing more-interoperable medical capabilities.

In INDOPACOM, a lack of consistent, multiyear funding has made it difficult for U.S. medical personnel to develop relationships with partner nations with an eye toward sustaining U.S. access and influence, but it has also limited their ability to increase regional trauma care and MEDEVAC capabilities that could be needed to support potential military operations or humanitarian disaster assistance missions. APRI, for example, only provides support for military-to-military contacts for a single year and is not consistently available; this has precluded components from sequencing projects and activities in a way that would maximize their

---

[147] Discussion with DoD official, November 6, 2020.

effectiveness and impact.[148] When O&M funds are used to support medical activities during exercises, they are not prioritized for building partner nation medical capacity or interoperability with more-capable partners. Overall, DoD officials in INDOPACOM told us that support provided to GHE activities by APRI and O&M exercises funds—the primary sources of GHE funding—does not allow for consecutive engagements and is not sufficient for meeting the operational readiness of the components or the GCC overall requirements.[149]

Indeed, similar challenges have affected GHE execution and planning across other GCCs. In EUCOM, medical planners revealed that the limited availability of funding has restricted the ability of service components to provide subject-matter expert exchanges and certification visits to support the development of NATO-standard Role 1 and Role 2 capabilities. Although medical planners have been able to provide more-focused support to Eastern European countries, they have not been able to provide the longer-term training and infrastructure support that many partners need.[150] One GHE stakeholder indicated that EUCOM has not been able to "crack the code" on obtaining funding for training and equipping for expeditionary medical capability among countries in the former Soviet Union.[151] EUCOM also has not been able to dedicate funding to conduct engagements with Western European countries to develop more-interoperable military medical support in the European theater.[152]

Our discussions with DoD officials also revealed that few EUCOM exercises include a medical training component, and service components are often unable to support partner requests for training across many health engagements. When specific requests from individual countries do receive support, they are one-off initiatives; this has made it difficult to expand efforts to build hospital capacity, develop aeromedical evacuation capabilities with additional partners, or execute a regional plan for building medical support over time.[153] According to one stakeholder assigned to the theater, GHE personnel have responded to this shortfall by organizing annual conferences to market GHE and its contributions to GCC priorities in an effort to increase the chances that future proposals will receive funding.[154] However, GHE is still not integrated into operational plans and is not prioritized as proposals for engagements continue to vie for funding with nonmedical security cooperation activities. In sum, although EUCOM maintains health-specific lines of effort, funding limitations continue to be a major barrier to taking advantage of

---

[148] Discussions with DoD official, January 26, 2021, and March 1, 2021.

[149] Discussion with U.S. defense officials, February 18, 2021.

[150] GHE stakeholders indicated that EDI funds, to date, have been used only for military-to-military visits and exchanges (discussion with U.S. defense officials, March 24, 2021).

[151] Discussion with U.S. defense official, August 11, 2020.

[152] DoD officials noted that they were not able to introduce a new health line of effort to include Western European countries, for example (discussion with U.S. defense official, August 11, 2020).

[153] Discussions with U.S. defense officials, August 11, 2020, and March 24, 2021.

[154] Discussion with U.S. defense officials, March 24, 2021.

opportunities to build medical capacity within key regions and to work with more-capable Western European partners to improve the availability of quality medical support in the event of a future military conflict.[155]

In CENTCOM, medical planners expressed very similar concerns regarding limited, one-year funding sources for GHE activities and the general inconsistency of funding. Interestingly, even when a country provided its own funds to support a trauma care facility, such as the UAE, planners found it challenging to engage U.S. medical personnel in providing necessary support. They noted that because the foreign military sale that funded the trauma center occurred outside the Joint Staff tasking process, it was not deemed necessary to provide manning or support.[156]

In the AFRICOM theater, short-term and inconsistent funding for GHE has limited the ability of the service components to build sustainable partner military medical capacities for disease surveillance, containment, and response. Funding limitations have also inhibited advancements in force protection across the region. Although some capacity-building support is provided through counterterrorism and peacekeeping operations programs, medical planners found it difficult to incorporate medical events within these programs and expressed frustration with the difficulty they face trying to employ one-year funding to conduct planned multiyear medical engagements. Service component personnel noted that the time and effort required to "dig" for short-term funding limits their ability to engage in effective capacity-building efforts.[157] Many GHE personnel in the theater are forced to rebuild portfolios each year as a result of one-year funding sources, which adds to the continuity challenge already made severe by the frequent rotation of GHE personnel into and out of the AFRICOM theater.

Many of above-mentioned funding-related challenges are also relevant to GHE in the SOUTHCOM theater. Short-term funding has limited the sustainment of public health initiatives, many of which are important to achieving objectives related to providing medical care helpful in maintaining access and influence in the region, as well as U.S. medical capabilities and readiness.[158] Limited funding has also restricted the ability of U.S. forces to fulfill partner military requests for U.S.-led GHE efforts: for example, building flight programs and sending a partner nation's military personnel to courses and trainings in the continental United States.[159]

Table 4.1 summarizes our findings in terms of the major differences in GHE sources of funding across the GCCs and the associated challenges that these funding limitations pose. It demonstrates that although each of the GCCs relies on different funding sources, they all face a common challenge of trying to implement GHE activities with limited, short-term funding. Most funding mechanisms are only able to support standalone engagements, as opposed to robust

---

[155] Discussion with U.S defense officials, August 11, 2020.

[156] Discussion with U.S. defense official, March 2, 2021.

[157] Discussions with U.S. defense officials, November 24, 2020, and March 15, 2021.

[158] Discussion with U.S. defense official, March 4, 2021.

[159] Discussion with U.S. defense official, March 25, 2021.

multiyear programs, and are often not prioritized for funding by the GCCs, DSCA, or the Office of the Secretary of Defense.

Table 4.1. GHE Funding Sources and Challenges Across the GCCs

GCC	Primary Funding Sources	Summary of Major Challenges
INDOPACOM	• APRI • OHDACA • O&M	• Short-term funding limits ability to build regional capabilities and sustain access • Medical events fall below "cut line" of theater priorities
EUCOM	• EDI • TCA	• Short-term funding limits ability to develop NATO-standard Role 1 and Role 2 capabilities • Lack of funding for infrastructure and training activities • Competition with nonmedical activities
CENTCOM	• TCA • FMS	• Inconsistent funding and timelines limit opportunities for engagement • Difficulties integrating FMS funding into GHE and developing trauma care facilities
AFRICOM	• PREACT • TSCTP • PEPFAR • APRRP	• Short-term and inconsistent funding limits ability to build sustainable partner capacity needed for disease containment and force protection • Misalignment between Title 10 and Title 22 funding cycles and processes
SOUTHCOM	• OHDACA • O&M	• Short-term funding limits sustainment of public health initiatives • Lack of resources for training U.S. medics • Failure to obtain Cooperative Threat Reduction designation leaves region without more-flexible DTRA funding

GHE Is Not Prioritized by the GCCs

Medical planners across the GCCs highlighted the difficulties they face when it comes to obtaining consistent funding to support GHE activities. These difficulties can largely be attributed to the inherent complexities of security cooperation and the fact that many GHE activities must compete for limited security cooperation resources that are designed for a variety of purposes. Although not all GHE activities are supported by security cooperation funding sources, those that are under GCC control are often limited in scope. In many cases, global health is considered a secondary objective for the use of these funds that are intended to provide humanitarian assistance, conduct counterterrorism operations, or increase U.S. access and influence.

More significantly, many stakeholders pointed out that most combatant commanders and J5 planners fail to prioritize funding for global health activities. Facing a great deal of competition for limited funds that commanders have available to allocate for security cooperation activities, GHE is not seen as critical to meeting operational requirements. In many cases, GHE activities are considered "nice to have" to help develop better relationships with partner nations, rather than "must-have" activities to ensure force protection or medical readiness. There is no direct link to operational plans or potential impact for GHE in terms of providing needed medical support to U.S. forces and avoiding casualties.

Several medical planners in INDOPACOM noted that the majority of GHE proposals for APRI funding are denied because they do not "make it above the cut line," as other activities are considered to be more important to achieving GCC objectives.[160] According to one former official, INDOPACOM received funding for only five of the 50 GHE-related proposals it submitted for funding each year, which they attributed to the fact that GHE is not considered to be aligned with the theater's operational lines of effort.[161] Other officials noted that the service components fail to consider medical activities as a priority for regional exercises, because these activities are rarely viewed as critical to achieving service readiness objectives.[162]

Similarly, medical planners in CENTCOM noted that proposals for GHE fail to compete well against other lines of effort because they are not considered to be critical to achieving the combatant commander's operational objectives.[163] The benefits of increasing trauma capacity and interoperability in the region did not appear to be a priority; in fact, one GHE stakeholder pointed out that medical is often "estranged" from GCC planning.[164] In SOUTHCOM, a GHE stakeholder noted that the combatant command was unable to recognize the operational benefits of providing U.S. medical training in remote areas and embedding medical personnel in local hospitals. This severely curtailed the ability of GHE proposals to compete effectively for OHDACA or global capacity-building funding available in the GCC.[165] In AFRICOM, medical activities are rarely prioritized by the combatant commander. Prior to 2020, medical and health engagements constituted only a small sliver of the security force assistance activities conducted for counterterrorism and peacekeeping.[166]

Global health engagements are rarely subject to assessment or evaluation and are not typically viewed through an operational lens by planners in the combatant commands (J5). In many cases, GHE activities are initiated at the country level and often are motivated by a desire to take advantage of opportunities to engage with willing partners to improve bilateral relationships, rather than a requirement to support U.S. medical readiness or force protection objectives.[167] As a result, GHE activities are not prioritized for security cooperation funding.

---

[160] Discussions with U.S. defense officials, January 7, 2021, and March 1, 2021.

[161] The official referenced past proposals partly because many APRI-funded activities were canceled in 2020 and 2021 because of the COVID-19 pandemic (discussions with U.S. defense officials, January 22, 2021, and March 1, 2021).

[162] Discussions with U.S. defense officials, February 4, 2021, and March 1, 2021.

[163] Discussions with U.S. defense officials, March 9, 2021.

[164] Discussions with U.S. defense officials, March 9, 2021.

[165] Discussion with U.S. defense official, March 4, 2021.

[166] AFRICOM, 2019.

[167] Discussions with DoD personnel, March 24, 2021.

Few officials outside the medical community advocate for GHE activities because GCC planners do not recognize their importance in supporting operational plans. This makes it difficult for GHE activities to vie for limited GCC funding or O&M exercise support. It also makes it difficult for GHE activity proposals to successfully compete for Section 333 partnership capacity-building funds.

Currently, medical planners have few means to support the building of military medical capacity in key regions of Europe, Africa, and the Pacific. They are also limited in their ability to develop the interoperable MEDEVAC and medical support capabilities with allies and partners that can play a critical role in maintaining the operational readiness of U.S. forces. GHE activities are generally not subject to assessment or evaluation; in most cases, GHE objectives are considered secondary or tertiary objectives for security cooperation activities and are not prioritized for support. The lack of dedicated funding sources for GHE and the short-term nature of funding further accentuate this challenge.

GHE Stakeholders Expressed the Need for Improved Funding Mechanisms to Support GHE Activities

During our discussions with GHE stakeholders, we asked them to describe the characteristics of an ideal funding source for GHE programs and activities going forward. Their answers varied but can be summarized into three options. First, some GHE stakeholders expressed the desire to have access to a multiyear funding source that would allow medical personnel to work with partner nations to enhance their medical capacity and interoperable medical capabilities according to theater demands. Second, some stakeholders advocated for a dedicated GHE fund that would create a "one-stop shop" for supporting medical engagements with partner nations.[168] Finally, others believed that it would be best to generate greater support for GHE-related activities through existing mechanisms for building partner capacity or interoperability.[169] However, as one official noted, GHE activities will not be prioritized for funding until "the line-side" (the operational components of DoD) view GHE as more than a soft-power tool and acknowledge the persistent and critical need for medical support for U.S. forces wherever they are deployed.[170] Therefore, GHE stakeholders stress that more-consistent GHE support will require more closely linking these types of engagements to theater requirements.

Moreover, several defense officials said that GHE should be described as being directly tied to meeting operational requirements for U.S. medical readiness and force protection. One official stated that "readiness is something everyone needs" and understands, noting that "GHE for U.S. readiness" could be the tagline for describing the value of GHE funding.[171] Another official said

---

[168] Discussions with DoD personnel, January 15, 2021; March 1, 2021; and March 29, 2021.

[169] Discussions with DoD personnel, January 22, 2021; February 26, 2021; March 3, 2021; and May 11, 2021.

[170] Discussions with DoD personnel, February 4, 2021.

[171] Discussions with DoD personnel, January 22, 2022.

that the purpose of GHE must be understood from the GCC commander's perspective as a means of enabling U.S. forces to be ready to conduct theater operations.[172]

DoD Stakeholders Indicated That There Was Insufficient Support for a Designated GHE Funding Source or Program of Record at This Time

Although many GHE planners recognize the need for more-consistent funding to support engagement with partner nations and see the potential benefits of having a designated source of funding for GHE, DoD officials acknowledged during a series of group conference calls that it will be difficult to establish such a dedicated source of funding, or what the DoD CBA referred to as a GHE "program of record" (i.e., similar to an acquisition program). Officials noted that DoD does not endorse requests for legislative relief—or new sources of congressional funding— if such activities can be conducted with internal DoD funds. As of this writing, DoD has not yet prioritized funding for any types of GHE activity. To illustrate this point, one official who participated in a group conference call said that "if the medical community can't articulate a reason for more funding, then DoD won't support a request to Congress."[173] Moreover, another official noted that a lack of support for a new source of GHE funding reflects the reality that the need for GHE as it is currently defined is not understood to be a high enough priority for DoD.[174] This gap could be addressed, according to several officials, by enhancing the broader understanding of the means through which GHE can address operational requirements.[175]

Recommendations

Link GHE to Theater and Global Planning and Reinforce the Importance of Assessment, Monitoring, and Evaluation

To ensure that GHE is effectively meeting combatant command requirements, medical personnel within the GCCs will need to work closely with their respective J5 planners. It will be critical for the J5 strategic planning staff to clarify their operational readiness requirements and potential needs for medical support. These operational demands can then shape GHE priorities. Each of the GCCs has different requirements, and it will be important to determine which medical support capabilities are most needed and where GHE should be targeted to have the greatest impact on U.S. operational readiness. Doing so will help determine the type of GHE activities that DoD should pursue and the most-critical allies and partners with whom the United States will need to work.

---

[172] Discussions with DoD personnel, September 7, 2021.

[173] Discussions with DoD officials, July 14, 2021.

[174] Discussions with DoD officials, July 14, 2021.

[175] Discussions with DoD officials, November 12, 2020; April 29, 2021; and July 14, 2021.

Using these operational requirements, the **GCCs should work with the Joint Staff and the Office of the Secretary of Defense's DASD for Global Partnerships (GP) to develop regionally specific GHE plans**. Coordination with the Joint Staff and the Office of the Secretary of Defense will ensure that GHE is prioritized as an operational requirement and incorporated into exercise planning, partnership capacity-building programs, and other security cooperation engagement efforts. Moreover, regional GHE plans can serve as a basis for tracking and assessing GHE activities over time to evaluate their effectiveness. GHE plans targeted to meeting GCC requirements for medical support are more likely to be prioritized for funding if they can demonstrate their value.

Further, **DASD/GP should consider ways to incorporate GHE into its security cooperation evaluation and learning agenda.** This would draw increased attention and resources toward conducting assessment, monitoring, and evaluation on medical- and health-related security cooperation activities on a regional and country basis. Such a move would help to inform future GHE funding decisions and strengthen linkages with the J5 community writ large. Specifically, evaluation results will help to inform the support base for GHE, strengthen the links with GCC plans, and make it easier for GHE to compete for funding. The analysis might even pave the way for a new source of dedicated funding that is targeted for GHE in the future.

The analysis and findings from GHE-focused strategic evaluations could help medical personnel at the GCC and service component level better articulate why GHE is needed, where it will be most beneficial in ensuring the health and safety of U.S. forces, and how it can improve the ability of U.S. forces to conduct current or future operations. It would require the drafting of a logic model (such as those used in designing significant security cooperation initiatives) that would include clearly stated GHE objectives that are directly linked to GCC operational requirements and demonstrate how these objectives are tied to GHE activities. It would then identify the expected outcomes for these activities and outline how progress toward meeting those outcomes would be measured. This would help to clarify not only what dedicated funding could be used for but also how its impact would be tracked and assessed.

Although there is consensus among GHE stakeholders on the need for more-consistent support for GHE activities to develop partner-nation medical capacity and interoperable medical capabilities, it will be difficult to obtain support for the establishment of a dedicated source of GHE funding (equivalent to a program of record) or other new funding sources without **more clearly demonstrating the link between GHE and U.S. GCC operational requirements,** as well as the potential savings that GHE activities might yield in terms of financial costs and the lives of U.S. forces. Support from the Joint Staff J5 and Congress would be required to pursue such an effort.

Thus, until GHE is better understood as meeting an operational imperative and directly supporting GCC objectives, it will be difficult to establish a case for creating a new, dedicated source of long-term support for GHE activities. Recognizing that this process may take time, we outline several ways that the military medical community could use existing funding sources to better meet combatant command objectives in the following recommendation.

Identify More-Consistent Sources of Support for GHE Through Existing Funding Mechanisms

To ensure that GHE activities receive more-consistent support, **DASD/GP should seek to better leverage existing security cooperation mechanisms while continuing to pursue dedicated GHE funding** to increase partner-nation capacity and capabilities for the purpose of enhancing medical support for U.S. forces. Given the diversity of theater requirements for force protection and medical readiness, it will be necessary to pursue several funding options. Moreover, it may be more effective to focus on using existing sources of funding until stakeholders can garner sufficient support to establish a dedicated GHE funding mechanism.

We describe four additional courses of action that DoD could take to better leverage existing funding mechanisms or to establish a new source of dedicated support for GHE. We outline some of the advantages and disadvantages of each option below and in Table 4.2.

Option 1: Better Utilize Current, Regionally Based Funding to Support GHE Activities

Better utilizing existing regionally based funding can be accomplished by designating GHE as a priority for funding within sources that are already being used to support some GHE activities. Options in this area could include using EDI or adding GHE as a line of effort to be funded under the Pacific Deterrence Initiative (PDI). Currently, EDI supports GHE military-to-military exchange visits that provide subject-matter expertise; if military medical support were to be recognized as a component of U.S. force posture in Europe, EDI funds might also support medical infrastructure in key locations. EDI could also fund military medical exercises with partners in the region. In the INDOPACOM theater, PDI was established as a budget display rather than a dedicated source of funding, and no PDI-related funds have supported GHE activities to date.[176] (Most GHE activities are supported by the APRI fund, which is limited to military-to-military exchanges.) However, PDI could similarly provide medical infrastructure support for Pacific nations if such support were deemed critical to improving the posture and capabilities of U.S. forces in the Indo-Pacific.[177]

Although the use of regional funds would be more effective for supporting GHE activities in Europe and the Pacific than in other regions, other options that draw on existing funds could be

---

[176] As of 2022, Congress had not established a dedicated appropriations account for PDI, and it was not part of DoD's Planning, Programming, Budgeting, and Execution cycle (Dustin Walker, "Show Me the Money: Boost the Pacific Deterrence Initiative," *War on the Rocks*, June 29, 2022).

[177] Congress authorized $7.1 billion for the PDI in the 2022 National Defense Authorization Act, $2.1 billion over DoD's budget request. The EDI received $570 million over DoD's budget request, bringing its total funding to about $4 billion. However, EDI will likely be expanded in light of the February 2022 Russian invasion of Ukraine (Andrew Eversden, "Pacific Deterrence Initiative Gets $2.1 Billion Boost in Final NDAA," *Breaking Defense*, December 7, 2021).

targeted more specifically elsewhere. In the CENTCOM region, for example, OCO funds could be targeted to support GHE activities aimed at improving regional trauma care facilities that could support U.S. forces. In regions such as SOUTHCOM, where humanitarian assistance is a more widely employed funding source, it may be possible to dedicate more funding for GHE through a Humanitarian Assistance Program. This option could address the need to build regional health infrastructure and could receive support if activities are explicitly linked to meeting U.S. force protection requirements as a critical secondary objective.

There are limitations to each of these options, however, in terms of both their scope and their predictability because they are often subject to internal competition for funding. According to U.S. defense officials, it is unlikely that DoD or Congress would support the fencing of designated funds for GHE.[178] Therefore, GHE support would have to be racked and stacked with other operational requirements, which could make it difficult to support long-term capacity-building efforts.

Option 2: Tap into Existing Training and Equipping Funds for GHE

Section 333 partnership capacity-building funds could provide enhanced support to GHE, if medical capacity-building is linked to a new humanitarian assistance mission area under consideration for the Section 333 authority. Similarly, GHE may receive more support if the development of health capacity is designated as institutional capacity-building under the Section 332 or 333 authorities. Medical capacity-building could also be designated as a potential source of Foreign Military Financing support or prioritized for future FMS cases.

These options would provide GCCs with direct support for BPC. However, even if the development of medical capacity is included among Section 333, Section 332, or Foreign Military Financing (FMF) objectives, it is unlikely that GHE would be prioritized within the existing competitive proposal process.

Option 3: Expand DoD's Authority to Use Defense Health Program Funds to Develop Partner Medical Capacity for the Purpose of Ensuring U.S. Force Protection

By expanding the use of DHP funding to support GHE activities aimed at developing partner-nation medical capacity, DoD could conduct more-targeted efforts to protect U.S. forces operating outside the continental United States, which would align with the Defense Health Agency's role as a combat support agency.[179] DHP funding could be tailored to GCC priorities and could support specific partner-nation facilities, such as blood banks or field hospitals, that could be used by U.S. forces to meet medical support needs in key regions.[180] Such funding

---

[178] Conference call with GHE stakeholders, September 7, 2021.

[179] As a combat support agency, the Defense Health Agency is responsible for providing or augmenting the medical capabilities of the combatant commands, the military services, federal partners, and partners and allies (DoD, Military Health System, "Combat Support," webpage, undated-a).

[180] Discussion with DoD official, May 11, 2021.

sources could be valuable in remote areas where U.S. forces may be stationed with few other sources of medical support, especially in the context of a contingency. To more closely link this effort to U.S. operational objectives, location selections could be informed by evolving plans to develop more-distributed bases through the concept of agile combat employment.

A DHP-supported GHE fund would allow the Joint Staff Surgeon to direct this support to the areas that are the most critical to ensuring the health and safety of U.S. forces globally. The fund would be able to cross service lines to provide funding jointly and could build on recent efforts to address the COVID-19 pandemic.[181] However, there may be internal competition for funding and a limit to the degree that DHP would be able to support a global effort, considering its own fiscal constraints.

Option 4: Designate Support for GHE Within the Service O&M Accounts for Medical Readiness

In fiscal year 2021, DHP has transferred the service medical readiness to the military departments to better meet U.S. operational requirements.[182] Medical readiness is now a service line item. It may be possible to designate or allow for funding for GHE activities from the service O&M accounts for the purpose of improving U.S. medical readiness. This could include conducting exercises and training with partner nations to develop interoperable tactical support and MEDEVAC capabilities. Such funding might also support embedded health care engagement teams in austere environments to ensure medical readiness and enhance interoperability for conducting expeditionary medical support. Moreover, such funds might provide support for the prepositioning of medical supplies or help develop fixed facilities for U.S. forces that could be critical to supporting medical operations in denied environments.[183] This type of fund would be global in nature but likely would be targeted to regions that are focused on contingency planning.

The use of service O&M funding for GHE would require buy-in from each of the services. Each would need to see the relevance of GHE to its medical readiness requirements. Competition for limited resources would be a major barrier. Yet service O&M funding would offer the most direct means of supporting medical readiness. U.S. defense officials indicated that it may be possible to use these funds for GHE activities that have a direct link to theater operational plans in critical regions.[184] Recognizing the potential implications of a conflict in Europe on U.S. medical readiness may also lead to greater support for working with allies and partners in this area. Nevertheless, further analysis will be required to understand the context in which medical

---

[181] Discussions with DoD official, November 12, 2020, and April 29, 2021.

[182] Office of the Under Secretary of Defense (Comptroller), *Defense Health Program: Fiscal Year (FY) 2021 Budget Estimates*, February 2020a, p. DHP-3.

[183] Discussions with DoD official, November 12, 2020, and April 29, 2021.

[184] Discussions with DoD official, November 12, 2020, and April 29, 2021.

readiness funds could be used to support GHE activities. Table 4.2 summarizes these four options.

Table 4.2. Analysis of Potential Courses of Action for Expanding Funding for GHE to Meet GCC Objectives

Course of Action	Flexibility	Scope of Activities	Competition for Funding	Source of Funding
Designate GHE support within regional funds	• Regionally specific • Could provide more-consistent support for capacity-building efforts, including infrastructure support	• May be limited to regions of potential high-end conflict • EDI or PDI with focus on force posture	• Internal competition for funding if GHE activities are not prioritized by GCCs or Congress	• No additional cost if within existing appropriation
Designate GHE support within existing training and equipping programs	• Global • Limited to training and equipping	• Limited by Section 333 mission areas, possibly extending to disaster response • May include limited number of FMF/FMS cases	• Highly selective Section 333 process • Limited FMF funding • FMF/FMS would be dependent, in part, on partner priorities	• Funding within existing Section 333
Expand DHP funding to include support for GHE for purpose of U.S. force health protection	• Global • Focused on force protection	• Military-to-military activities with partner-nation medical personnel	• May be internal competition over specific regions or countries receiving support	• Would require funding from DHP budget
Allow for GHE to be supported by service O&M funding for medical readiness	• Global • Focus on medical readiness • Could include infrastructure support	• Capability development activities: military-to-military training, exercises, and possible prepositioning of medical supplies	• Prioritization likely given to regions focused on contingency planning (Pacific, Europe, Middle East)	• Would require funding from service O&M accounts

Conclusion

Our research suggests that the most optimal initial course of action would likely involve pursuing efforts to better use existing funds: particularly, regional funding mechanisms that are tied to improving U.S. force posture. Efforts to draw on EDI and PDI to support GHE activities in Europe and the Pacific appear to be the most promising, given the links between GHE

47

activities and U.S. strategic objectives of (1) ensuring the readiness of U.S. forces and (2) serving as an effective deterrent to adversaries. EDI and PDI funds could be employed to build more-resilient medical support capabilities with allies and partners that are critical to achieving U.S. integrated deterrence goals.

At the same time, we also recommend pursuing new funding sources to provide dedicated support for medical readiness. Although DHP may be more effective in addressing force health protection issues, the O&M fund would likely support a wide range of medical readiness exercises and training that could be critical to developing interoperability with allies and partners. Currently, there is no dedicated funding to support the combined medical capabilities that may be necessary in a future contingency. Such a fund could also help to address potential medical logistics shortages, which were not addressed in this report, and could prove critical to maintaining U.S. operational readiness in a conflict with a near-peer adversary.

With greater recognition of the potential demand for combat casualty care in a future conflict, DoD and Congress might prioritize GHE for funding.[185] As we note above, further analysis can help clarify how the newly established readiness fund could support GHE or lead to a separate designated fund for GHE activities with a separate congressional allocation.

Each of the funding options we discussed will require close coordination between medical planners within the Office of the Joint Staff Surgeon, command surgeons, and J5 strategic planning staff across the GCCs and the Defense Health Agency, as well as OASD Health Affairs, to ensure that any new mechanism effectively meets U.S. operational objectives. It will also be necessary to engage the interagency community that is involved with GHE to ensure that GHE is integrated into the broader U.S. approach to global health. The military medical community will need to ensure that it focuses on its niche for engaging with partner military medical forces but also will need to contribute to broader global health security efforts. In fact, many of the capacity-building efforts and medical readiness exercises that fall under the scope of GHE may have secondary benefits for meeting Global Health Security Agenda goals.

It will also be important for OASD Health Affairs to remain engaged with the DoD Comptroller, Office of General Counsel, and congressional liaisons to determine what options are feasible and whether and how they might be pursued, including obtaining the necessary support. OASD Health Affairs will also need to continue to frame GHE as an operational imperative to ensure that U.S. forces have the necessary medical support in the face of a global pandemic, a humanitarian disaster, or a potential conflict with a near-peer adversary. Until the medical community can demonstrate the value of engaging with allies and partners in the domain of health and medical activities—and can show how this engagement is integral to meeting current and future strategic requirements—it is unlikely that GHE will receive dedicated resources.

---

[185] Thomas, 2021.

Finally, we highlight that any courses of action taken to increase funding for GHE should be designed with an assessment framework that connects activities to theater operational and strategic objectives and evaluates program effectiveness in meeting operational requirements for force protection and medical readiness over time. To adequately assess progress, it will be necessary to employ more-comprehensive information technology (IT) support to track ongoing and future GHE activities. Moreover, for both current and future GHE efforts to be successful in meeting U.S. objectives, it will be critical to ensure that U.S. military medical professionals and security cooperation planners receive adequate education and training. These two topics—IT and education and training—are the topics of the two companion reports in this series.[186]

---

[186] Marquis et al., 2023; and Vedula et al., 2023.

Appendix A. GHE-Related Funding Sources 101

This appendix provides an overview of the major sources of funding that have been used to support GHE activities. Although it does not include all possible funding sources, it includes those funding sources that were mentioned during our meetings with GHE stakeholders and the funding sources that were mentioned in secondary sources as being used to support GHE activity. Table A.1 provides a brief description of each funding type, the relevant authority, and the time frame for the obligation and expenditure of funds.

Table A.1. GHE-Related Funding Sources

Funding Mechanism	Description	Related Authority	Funding Time Frame
DoD-Managed and DoD-Executed Programs			
Asia Pacific Regional Initiative (APRI)	• Congressional appropriation for INDOPACOM to execute theater security cooperation activities (e.g., humanitarian assistance, U.S. personnel costs)[a] • APRI is funded under Navy O&M, $14 million in FY 2021 and $11 million in FY 2022.[b] • APRI may be used for military-to-military contacts; it cannot be used for training and equipping or infrastructure support for partners. • Funding is available for individual events in a single fiscal year. • GHE activities are limited to exchanges and public health outreach.	• Public Law 115-409, FY 2018	• Single-year obligation and expenditure
Biological Threat Reduction Program (BTRP)	• Program within DoD's Cooperative Threat Reduction program, designed to address WMD challenges; it is not security cooperation • BTRP supports activities to reduce the proliferation of biological weapons and activities to facilitate detection and reporting of pathogens.[c] • BTRP is funded through annual appropriation, which was anticipated to be $127 million in FY 2021.[d] • In response to the COVID-19 pandemic, BTRP appears to have received additional funding as part of U.S. global health security efforts, for a total of $225 million in FY 2021.[e] • Three-year funding, with allowance to complete projects within five years, but limited to biosecurity, biosafety, and biosurveillance • Global program managed by DTRA, separate from the GCCs; South American countries are not designated for BTRP support • GHE activities include exercises, tabletop exercises, and OneHealth workshops.	• U.S. Code, Title 50, Section 3711	• Funding executed over a three-year period, with allowance to complete projects within five years

51

Funding Mechanism	Description	Related Authority	Funding Time Frame
Combatant Commander's Initiative Fund (CCIF)	• Fund allowing the Chairman of the Joint Chiefs of Staff to support U.S. training, contingencies, selected operations, command and control, joint exercises, humanitarian assistance, military education, personnel expenses, force protection, and joint warfighting capabilities • Fund is intended to enable U.S. forces "to act quickly to support Combatant Commanders . . . to solve emergent challenges and unforeseen contingency requirements."[f] • GCC funds are only available to "support a single, identified project and are not a source of funding for a continuing project."[g] • CCIF was used in the past for pandemic preparedness efforts.[h]	• U.S. Code, Title 10, Section 166a[i]	• One-year funding for single, identified projects
European Deterrence Initiative (EDI)	• EDI is a congressionally authorized initiative to enhance U.S. deterrence posture, increase the readiness and responsiveness of U.S. forces in Europe, and support the collective security of NATO allies.[j] — EDI lines of effort include Increased Presence, Exercises and Training, Enhanced Prepositioning, Improved Infrastructure, and Building Partnership Capacity. • $4.5 billion in funding in FY 2021; $3.7 million requested in FY 2022[k] • EDI support for GHE has been limited to one-time military-to-military events with partner nations. Infrastructure support has only been provided to the U.S. Army for prepositioned stock and for Air Force health services equipment. To date, Ukraine is the only country to receive equipment, training, logistics support, and supplies.[l]	• Public Law 115-91, Section 1273 (2018 National Defense Authorization Act)	• Until FY 2022, EDI has been funded through DoD's OCO account, which is appropriated annually. • OCO-funded programs are not part of the Future Years Defense Program and are generally planned for one year at a time[m]

52

Funding Mechanism	Description	Related Authority	Funding Time Frame
Humanitarian and Civic Assistance (HCA)	• Funding is authorized for humanitarian activities conducted in conjunction with DoD operations and exercises in a foreign country.[n] • U.S. personnel may provide support to a foreign nation's local populace, but the primary purpose must be to enable DoD activities.[o] • HCA support cannot be provided directly or indirectly to any individual, group, or organization engaged in military activity. • HCA receives specifically appropriated O&M funds for de minimus (incidental) activities. Average annual global expenditure is $5 million to $8 million.[p] • GHE activities include medical, dental, and veterinary care in rural areas in conjunction with U.S. exercises for a limited time (mostly, one-time events). Can be done alongside partner-nation forces, nongovernmental organizations, etc.	• U.S. Code. Title 10, Section 401	• One-year funding

Overseas Humanitarian, Disaster, and Civic Aid (OHDACA)	• Congressional appropriation for humanitarian assistance activities[q]
	• Funds are appropriated annually but are available for two-year periods.[r]
	• OHDACA funds support five Title 10 authorized programs, including
	  – Humanitarian Assistance (HA)
	  – Humanitarian Mine Action (HMA)
	  – Foreign Disaster Relief (FDR)
	  – Nonlethal Excess Property (EP)
	  – Funded Transportation Program (FTP)
	  – Denton Space-Available Transportation Program.[s]
	• Total OHDACA funding is approximately $105 million per year.[t]
	• OHDACA support can only be provided to civilians. Medical support is intended for unique, time-sensitive capabilities that cannot be provided by other agencies.
	• Humanitarian assistance may include health-focused projects, including hospital and clinic construction, medical supplies, and public health assessments.
		• Title 10, Sections 2561 (HA), 407 (HMA), 404 (FDR), 2557 (EP), and 402 (Denton)	• Funds appropriated annually but available for two-year period

53

Funding Mechanism	Description	Related Authority	Funding Time Frame
Section 333 (Train and Equip)	• Section 333 is a security cooperation authority that allows DoD to build the capacity of foreign security partners to address emergent threats. • Training and equipment may be provided for the following activities: — Counterterrorism, Counter-WMD, Counter-illicit Drugs, Counter Transnational Crime, Maritime and Border Security, Military Intelligence, Air Domain Awareness, Cyberspace Security, or International Coalition Operations.[u] • Section 333 funding is allocated by Congress ($350 million in FY 2022) and managed by the Office of the Secretary of Defense. • Proposals for Section 333 supports must be submitted by the GCCs and undergo a competitive annual selection process. • Section 333 funding may have been used to support medical efforts tied to maritime defense and border security.[v]	• U.S. Code, Title 10, Section 333	• Funds are appropriated annually and may be expended over two years (or within two years of date that equipment or training is delivered)[w]
State Partnership Program (SPP)	• SPP is a DoD security cooperation program managed and administered by the National Guard Bureau and coordinated by the GCCs.[x] • The National Guard Bureau maintains 85 partnerships with 93 nations and conducts about 1,000 events annually.[y] — Partnerships are concentrated in Eastern Europe, where SPP was established in 1991. • Funding is provided by the National Guard Bureau for personnel and allowances; travel costs are covered through TCA, WIF, or other security cooperation programs. • Military medical is one of several focus areas of SPP, but most medical activities are limited to one-time events.[z] • GHE-related activities include subject-matter expert exchanges and training.[aa]	• U.S. Code, Title 10, Sections 168, 311, 312, 321, 341, 345[bb]	• Variety of one-year funding sources: e.g., TCA and WIF

54

Funding Mechanism	Description	Related Authority	Funding Time Frame
Traditional Combatant Command Activities (TCA)	• Funds available for combatant commanders to support regional security activities. • Funding is provided to GCCs through service O&M appropriations.[cc] • Activities include military liaison teams, traveling contact teams, state partnership programs, regional conferences and seminars, unit exchanges, staff assistance and assessment visits, joint and combined exercise observers, and bilateral staff talks, mostly for single events.[dd] • TCA may be used for GHE military-to-military activities but not for capacity-building.	• U.S. Code, Title 10, Sections 166a and 312	• One-year funding for single, identified projects
Wales Initiative Fund (WIF)	• Prior to 2021, WIF was an annual appropriation supporting defense reform efforts and institutional capacity-building with 16 Eastern European and Central Asian countries in the NATO Partnership for Peace program.[ee] • WIF was used to support exchanges, exercises, and workshops supporting NATO interoperability. • WIF was previously known as the Warsaw Initiative Fund. • Most activities WIF supported are now supported by the Security Cooperation Programs Account and regional centers, which fund defense institution-building, military-to-military contacts, payment of expenses to attend bilateral or regional conferences, and payment of training and exercise expenses.[ff]	• U.S. Code, Title 10, Sections 311, 312, 321, 332	• Annual appropriation, one-year funding

55

Funding Mechanism	Description	Related Authority	Funding Time Frame
Defense Health Program (DHP)	• DHP is a sub-account under the O&M account that funds military health system functions for U.S. forces; it is not a security cooperation fund. • Activities include health care delivery in military treatment facilities; TRICARE; certain medical readiness activities and expeditionary medical capabilities; education and training programs; research, development, test, and evaluation; management and headquarters activities; facilities sustainment; procurement; and civilian and contract personnel.[gg] • DHP O&M funds were $34 billion in FY 2021.[hh] • DHP supports professional military education programs through USUHS. • However, DHP funds do not support partner capacity-building efforts.[ii] • Research activities are supported through a grant mechanism by which DoD funds (e.g., Army Medical Research Acquisition Activity funds) are provided to the Henry M. Jackson Foundation and then distributed over multiple years.[jj]	• DHP account established via U.S. Code, Title 10, Section 1100[kk]	• One-year funding (although funding has been transferred to the Henry M. Jackson Foundation for the Advancement of Military Medicine to extend funding for USUHS)
State Department–Managed Programs			
African Peacekeeping Rapid Response Partnership (APRRP)	• Initiative to build international peacekeeping capacity in six nations: civil and military security forces to rapidly deploy and respond to crisis through the African Union and United Nations[ll] • APRRP funding is provided through Title 22 PKO authority • Most APRRP funding is linked to larger PKO activities and is not designed for building medical capacity. • However, the APRRP medical component has trained partner nations to develop capabilities to rapidly deploy and sustain field hospitals: United Nations–designated Level 2 hospitals that can provide primary and emergency surgical care to troops on the ground.[mm] • APRRP has also provided support for a Medical Modeling and Simulation Center and for medical planner courses to partners.[nn]	• U.S. Code, Title 22, Section 2348[oo]	• OCO-supported program, established as a three- to five-year program but subject to annual appropriations

56

Funding Mechanism	Description	Related Authority	Funding Time Frame
Foreign Military Sales (FMS)	• FMS is a security assistance program that allows foreign governments and international organizations to acquire U.S. defense articles and training through the DoD acquisition system.[pp] • Department of State manages FMS; DoD administers FMS • Eligible countries may purchase defense articles and services with their national funds or through U.S. Foreign Military Financing.[qq] • The UAE used FMS in a GHE-related case to support its Trauma, Burn, and Rehabilitative Medicine center; Croatia purchased two UH-60M Black Hawk helicopters for MEDEVAC through FMS.[rr]	• U.S. Code, Title 22, Section 2751, Arms Export Control Act, as amended	• FMS are partner-nation funded
Global Peace Operations Initiative (GPOI)	• GPOI is a State Department–managed initiative to strengthen international capacity and capabilities to execute United Nations and regional peace operations. • GPOI provides training, equipment, and advisory assistance to 35 partner countries. • Medical education and training are among the many enabling capabilities that GPOI can support.[ss] • Most medical engagements are only a secondary objective for GPOI activities.	• U.S. Code, Title 22, Section 2348[tt]	• Established as a five-year program, funding allocated to State Department annually
International Military Education and Training (IMET)	• IMET is a security assistance program managed by the State Department that provides grants for military education and training for foreign military personnel. • IMET is primarily used for professional military education and, by exception, for technical training. It is generally used for tuition expenses. • IMET funding is appropriated annually ($113 million in FY 2021).[uu] • Expanded-IMET (E-IMET) is a subcategory of IMET focused on specific issues including defense institution-building, military justice and human rights, responsible resourcing and budgets, and civilian control of the military.[vv]	• U.S. Code, Title 22, Sections 2347– 2347(d)	• Funds appropriated annually for single-year, individual education and training events

57

Funding Mechanism	Description	Related Authority	Funding Time Frame
Partnership for Regional East Africa Counterterrorism (PREACT)	• PREACT is a security assistance program for building partner military, law enforcement, and civil capacity to counter terrorism in East Africa.[ww] • PREACT, which is managed and administered by the State Department, derives funding from various foreign assistance accounts, including PKO.[xx] • DoD largely implements activities under PKO, which allows for training and equipping of partner-nation military forces. • PREACT medical activities have included combat medical training, but medical activities are often one-time events and are secondary to primary objectives.[yy]	• U.S. Code, Title 22, Section 2348	• Appropriated annually through State Department PKO account
President's Emergency Plan for AIDS Relief (PEPFAR)	• PEPFAR is a program managed by the Department of State for HIV/AIDS response and prevention.[zz] • Funding is provided through the DHP account.[aaa] • The DoD HIV/AIDS Prevention Program is the military implementing arm for PEPFAR, which assists "foreign military partners with the development and implementation of culturally focused, military-specific HIV/AIDS prevention, care, and treatment programs in more than 55 countries around the globe."[bbb] • AFRICOM has used PEPFAR to work with partner-nation militaries, limited to HIV/AIDS-related issues.	• U.S. Code, Title 22, Chapter 32, Foreign Assistance Act • Public Law 108–25, U.S. Leadership Against HIV/AIDS, Tuberculosis and Malaria Act of 2003 • Public Law 110–293, The Tom Lantos and Henry J. Hyde U.S. Global Leadership Against HIV/AIDS PEPFAR Extension Act of 2018[ccc]	• Appropriated annually through the Department of State; programmed through DHP account, which requires one-year obligations
Trans-Sahara Counterterrorism Partnership (TSCTP)	• TSCTP is a State Department–managed program to build partner capacity to counter violent extremism in North and West Africa and is jointly implemented by the State Department, DoD, and the U.S. Agency for International Development.[ddd] • TSCTP receives dedicated funding from several sources, including PKO.[eee] • TSCTP has supported humanitarian assistance efforts through Medical Civic Action Programs and Veterinary Civic Action Programs, but these events must be connected to counterterrorism objectives.[fff]	• U.S. Code, Title 22, Section 2348	• Appropriated annually through State Department PKO account

NOTE: FY = fiscal year; PKO = peacekeeping operations; WMD = weapons of mass destruction.
[a] The APRI was introduced in Public Law 111-118, Department of Defense Appropriations Act, 2010; Section 8094, December 19, 2009. It was most recently amended in Public Law 117-103, Consolidated Appropriations Act, 2022; Section 8042, Humanitarian Assistance, March 15, 2022.

Funding Mechanism	Description	Related Authority	Funding Time Frame

b Congress increased funding for APRI from $10 million in FY 2018 to $14 million in FY 2021, then decreased funding to $11 million in FY 2022 (Defense Security Cooperation University, 2020, p. 123; and Public Law 117-103, 2022).

c Defense Security Cooperation Agency, "Updates to the Program Codes for the Global Peacekeeping Operations Initiative (GPOI), Peacekeeping Operations (PKO) and Peacekeeping Operations African Peacekeeping Rapid Response Partnership (PKO/APRRP) Programs, DSCA Policy 19-41 [E-Change 444]," memorandum to the Deputy Assistant Secretary of the Army for Defense Exports and Cooperation, Deputy Assistant Secretary of the Navy for International Programs, and Deputy Under Secretary of the Air Force for International Affairs, September 23, 2019a; and U.S. Code, Title 50, Section 3711, Authority to Carry Out Department of Defense Cooperative Threat Reduction Program.

d Defense Security Cooperation Agency, 2019a; and Office of the Under Secretary of Defense (Comptroller), "Fiscal Year (FY) 2021 Budget Estimates: Operation and Maintenance, Defense-Wide, Cooperative Threat Reduction Program," February 2020c.

e Kaiser Family Foundation, "Breaking Down the U.S. Global Health Budget by Program Area," fact sheet, September 2022, p. 18.

f Office of the Under Secretary of Defense (Comptroller), "Fiscal Year (FY) 2021 Budget Estimates: Operation and Maintenance, Defense-Wide, The Joint Staff," February 2020d.

g Defense Security Cooperation University, Security Cooperation Management, 42nd ed., 2022, Ch. 17.

h U.S. Government Accountability Office, Influenza Pandemic: DOD Combatant Commands' Preparedness Efforts Could Benefit from More Clearly Defined Roles, Resources, and Risk Mitigation, GAO-07-696, June 2007.

i U.S. Code, Title 10, Section 166a, Combatant Commands: Funding Through the Chairman of Joint Chiefs of Staff.

j EDI was known as the European Reassurance Initiative when it was first initiated in 2014 (EUCOM, undated; quoted in Belkin and Kaileh, 2021).

k Office of the Under Secretary of Defense (Comptroller), 2020b, p. 2.

l Office of the Under Secretary of Defense (Comptroller), 2020b, pp. 18–19.

m As an OCO-funded program that relied on annual congressional appropriations, EDI was not included in DoD's Future Years Defense Program, which includes projected funding over five years (Belkin and Kaileh, 2021). Starting in FY 2022, EDI funding transitioned from the former OCO budget to the base budget.

n Department of Defense Instruction 2205.02, 2017.

o Joint Publication 3-29, Foreign Humanitarian Assistance, Joint Chiefs of Staff, May 14, 2019, p. I-10.

p Defense Security Cooperation University, 2020, p. 108.

q Defense Security Cooperation Agency, "Overseas Humanitarian, Disaster, and Civic Aid (OHDACA)," webpage, undated-b.

r Defense Security Cooperation Agency, undated-b.

s Defense Security Cooperation Agency, "Fiscal Year (FY) 2021 Budget Estimates: Operation and Maintenance, Defense-Wide, Overseas Humanitarian, Disaster, and Civic Aid," February 2020.

t Defense Security Cooperation Agency, 2020.

u U.S. Code, Title 10, Section 333.

v Discussion with U.S. defense officials, February 18, 2021.

w U.S. Code, Title 10, Section 333.

x DoD, The State Partnership Program: FY2015 Report to Congress, December 2016.

y National Guard, "State Partnership Program," fact sheet, undated.

z National Guard, undated.

aa Andrew Jackson, "Guam, Hawaii Share COVID Best Practices with the Philippines," National Guard, December 10, 2020; and Jesse Manzano, "Florida Guard Partners with Guyana to Boost Medical Readiness," National Guard, March 9, 2020.

bb Center for Army Lessons Learned, Security Cooperation and the State Partnership Program, October 2018.

cc Joint Publication 1-06, Financial Management in Joint Operations, Joint Chiefs of Staff, January 11, 2018.

dd Joint Publication 1-06, 2018, p. E-2.

ee Office of the Under Secretary of Defense (Comptroller), 2021.

ff Defense Security Cooperation University, 2021, p. 167; and Office of the Under Secretary of Defense (Comptroller), 2021.

gg Mendez, 2021.

Funding Mechanism	Description	Related Authority	Funding Time Frame

hh Mendez, 2021.

ii Center for Global Health Engagement, "2020 Annual Report," 2020; and Office of the Under Secretary of Defense (Comptroller), 2020a.

jj Cause IQ, undated.

kk U.S. Code, Title 10, Section 1100.

ll APRRP is targeted to Ethiopia, Ghana, Rwanda, Senegal, Tanzania, and Uganda to maintain forces and equipment that are ready to deploy to United Nations and African Union peacekeeping missions (AFRICOM, 2019; and U.S. Department of State, "U.S. Peacekeeping Capacity Building Assistance," fact sheet, May 27, 2022).

mm Sarah Marshall, "Global Health Engagement: The African Peacekeeping Rapid Response Partnership," *The Pulse*, Uniformed Services University blog, March 5, 2018.

nn Charles W. Beadling, "AFRICOM Health Engagement and Security: Beyond Hearts and Minds," Uniformed Services University of the Health Sciences, June 20, 2017; Uniformed Services University, "Department of Defense Global Health Engagement," briefing, undated; and U.S. Embassy in Rwanda, "Handover Ceremony of the AMEP Medical Modeling and Simulation Project," February 7, 2016.

oo Defense Security Cooperation Agency, 2019a.

pp Defense Security Cooperation Agency, "Foreign Military Sales (FMS)," webpage, undated.

qq Defense Security Cooperation University, 2022, Ch. 5, p. 5-1.

rr Discussions with U.S. military and defense officials; and Defense Security Cooperation Agency, "Croatia—UH-60M Black Hawk Helicopters," Transmittal No. 19-72, October 30, 2019b.

ss U.S. Department of State, "Key Topics—Office of Global Programs and Initiatives," webpage, undated-a.

tt The GPOI was established in 2004 as a five-year program to build foreign military capabilities to perform peacekeeping operations. Funding is requested under the State Department's PKO account, then obligated to DoD (Defense Security Cooperation Agency, 2019a; and Nina M. Serafino, *The Global Peace Operations Initiative: Background and Issues for Congress*, Congressional Research Service, June 11, 2009).

uu Defense Security Cooperation University, 2021.

vv Defense Security Cooperation University, 2021.

ww U.S. Department of State Bureau of Counterterrorism, "Programs and Initiatives," webpage, undated.

xx Other funding sources include the Economic Support Fund, International Narcotics Control and Law Enforcement Affairs, and Nonproliferation, Antiterrorism, Demining, and Related Programs. DoD activities are supported by PKO funds (U.S. Government Accountability Office, *Combating Terrorism: State Department Can Improve Management of East Africa Program*, GAO-14-502, June 2014a).

yy U.S. Senate, *Department of Defense Authorization for Appropriations for Fiscal Year 2018 and the Future Years Defense Program*, hearing before the Senate Committee on Armed Services, U.S. Government Publishing Office, 2020.

zz U.S. Department of State, "The United States President's Emergency Plan for AIDS Relief," webpage, undated-b.

aaa U.S. Government Accountability Office, *President's Emergency Plan for Aids Relief: State Should Improve Data Quality and Assess Long-Term Resource Needs*, GAO-21-374, May 2021, p. 6.

bbb Defense Health Agency, "Department of Defense HIV/AIDS Prevention Program," webpage, undated.

ccc Kellie Moss and Jennifer Kates, "PEPFAR Reauthorization: Side-by-Side of Legislation over Time," Kaiser Family Foundation, January 29, 2019.

ddd U.S. Department of State Bureau of Counterterrorism, undated.

eee The TSCTP program also receives funding from Development Assistance; Nonproliferation, Demining, and Related Programs; Economic Support Fund; and International Narcotics Control and Law Enforcement (U.S. Government Accountability Office, *Combating Terrorism: U.S. Efforts in Northwest Africa Would Be Strengthened by Enhanced Program Management*, GAO-14-518, June 2014b).

fff Lesley Anne Warner, *The Trans Sahara Counter Terrorism Partnership: Building Partner Capacity to Counter Terrorism and Violent Extremism*, CNA, March 2014, p. 50.

Appendix B. GCC GHE Priorities and Activities

Tables B.1, B.2, and B.3 provide a summary of the main GHE programs and activities across the five GCCs, broken down by service component. Table B.4 provides a summary of the Air Force components' primary GHE priorities and activities across each GCC. In our research, we found that theater priorities varied across each area of responsibility, with INDOPACOM, EUCOM, and CENTCOM focusing primarily on operational and contingency planning and AFRICOM and SOUTHCOM GHE efforts focused more on maintaining regional stability, access, and influence. GHE activities across the GCCs varied accordingly and contributed to increasing interoperability with partners and enhancing partner capacity via expeditionary medical and trauma care, disease containment, and other efforts.

Table B.1. INDOPACOM GHE Programs and Activities

Component	Major GHE Programs and Activities
PACAF	• Operation PACIFIC ANGEL (subject-matter expert exchanges related to infectious diseases, biosurveillance) – Medical and dental civic action programs • Exercise COPE NORTH (expeditionary medicine training with Australia and Japan) • BPC programs in aerospace medicine • BPC in patient movement, aeromedical evacuation
USARPAC	• USARPAC Protection Symposium (trauma care, MEDEVAC capabilities) • Subject-matter expert exchanges related to trauma care, public health, force health protection, biopreparedness
PACFLT	• PACIFIC PARTNERSHIP annual military exercise • U.S. Naval Medical Research Unit Two (infectious diseases) • Partner trauma training to support interoperability • BPC in critical care for operational medicine (shipboard military medical care)
MARFORPAC	• Marine Expeditionary Unit medically focused operations • PACIFIC PARTNERSHIP annual military exercise • Tactical-level health engagements during bilateral training exercises

Table B.2. EUCOM and CENTCOM GHE Programs and Activities

Component	Major GHE Programs and Activities
EUCOM	
USAFE	• Role 1 and Role 2 MEDEVAC certification (15 countries in former Soviet Union) • NATO, U.S., and partner-nation interoperability for combat casualty care • BPC for medical logistics, MEDEVAC, public health, force health • Various exercises (e.g., VIGOROUS WARRIOR)
U.S. Naval Forces Europe	• Various activities to promote interoperability (e.g., surgical trauma exchanges) • Tactical Combat Casualty Care course
CENTCOM	
AFCENT	• National trauma centers in Tier 1 partners • Defense Institute for Medical Operations courses • Train-Advise-Assist missions • BPC in aeromedical evacuation, trauma care

Table B.3. AFRICOM and SOUTHCOM GHE Programs and Activities

Component	Major GHE Programs and Activities
AFRICOM	
U.S. Air Forces Africa	• BPC in aerial patient movement, combat casualty care, CASEVAC • BPC in medical logistics • African Partnership Outbreak Response Alliance (disease containment)
U.S. Naval Forces Europe-Africa	• Military-to-military exchanges related to tactical combat casualty care, shipboard medicine, preventive medicine • APRRP: training and equipment for deployable hospital units • Africa Malaria Task Force • Pandemic response engagements (e.g., with the United Kingdom)
SOUTHCOM	
AFSOUTH	• BPC in patient movement • Tactical combat casualty care

Table B.4. GHE Across U.S. Air Force Component Commands

Component	Air Force GHE Priorities	Air Force Primary Activities
PACAF	• Partner interoperability • BPC for great-power competition • Increased focus on force health protection	• Regional patient movement and evacuation capabilities • Aerospace medicine • Biosurveillance
USAFE	• Deterrence • NATO support • Medical readiness for contingency • Force health protection	• Role 1 and Role 2 standard operating procedures for NATO certification • Aero evacuation capabilities
AFCENT	• Partner interoperability • Partner medical military capability • Readiness for ongoing operations	• Train-Advise-Assist • MEDEVAC capabilities • Trauma care • Role 2 medical facilities
U.S. Air Forces Africa	• Strengthen partner networks • Support to partners in Sahel and Lake Chad regions	• Partner patient movement and evacuation capabilities • Medical logistics • Infectious disease containment
AFSOUTH	• Humanitarian assistance and disaster relief • U.S. force readiness through public health • Partner capacity-building	• Partner patient movement capabilities • Trauma care • Vaccine distribution

SOURCE: Features information from GHE stakeholder discussions.

63

Appendix C. List of Organizations Involved in Discussions

Combatant Command Health Personnel Surgeon Offices

- AFRICOM
- CENTCOM
- EUCOM
- INDOPACOM
- SOUTHCOM
- SOCOM
- U.S. Transportation Command[187]

Air Components and Others

- USAFE-AFAFRICA Command Surgeon
- AFAFRICA GHE personnel
- AFCENT Command Surgeon and GHE personnel
- USAFE GHE personnel
- PACAF Command Surgeon and GHE personnel
- AFSOUTH GHE personnel
- Air Force Special Operations Command Surgeon
- U.S. Naval Forces Europe-Africa GHE personnel
- U.S. Special Operations Command South GHE personnel

INDOPACOM Components

- USARPAC
- PACFLT
- MARFORPAC
- PACAF Surgeon General and GHE Chief
- PACAF A5I (International Affairs)

Services and Health Agencies

- Navy Bureau of Medicine and Surgery
- Air Force Medical Service
- Army Medical Department
- U.S. Marine Corps Health Services
- Defense Health Agency

---

[187] Many discussions with Surgeon General and Command Surgeon offices included GHE personnel from these combatant commands. Our discussions included both officers and enlisted personnel.

- Defense Health Agency Veterinary Service
- Defense Institute for Medical Operations
- USUHS Center for Global Health Engagement
- DTRA
- Center for Excellence in Disaster Management and Humanitarian Assistance
- National Guard SPP

Other

- Joint Staff
- Office of the Assistant Secretary of Defense for Special Operations/Low-Intensity Conflict
- Office of the Secretary of Defense Comptroller
- DSCA, General Council
- Global Health Security Agenda
- Office of the Assistant Secretary of Defense for Health Affairs

Appendix D. Discussion Protocol

GLOBAL HEALTH ENGAGEMENT – IMPROVING SUPPORT TO COMBATANT COMMANDS

Discussion Protocol

INTRODUCTION

Thank you for taking the time to speak with us. RAND is conducting a study for the Office of the Assistant Secretary of Defense for Health Affairs (OASD/HA) that serves as a follow-on to the 2018 GHE Capability Based Assessment. OASD/HA has asked us to assess Global Health Engagement (GHE) education and training, technology platforms, and funding mechanisms to help DoD synchronize GHE training and education and enable long-term GHE capability development for the Combatant Commands (CCMDs). Our project monitor in the Health Affairs office is Dr. Chris Daniel, the senior advisor for Global Health Engagement.

We selected you in consultation with our sponsor because of your experience in the global health engagement field. Although we believe your insights will be quite valuable, you are of course free to decline to participate in the discussion, decline to answer any question, and to provide the level of detail you feel is appropriate.

BACKGROUND QUESTIONS

Would you please indicate the major DoD (or other USG or non-USG) organization you currently belong to (e.g., OSD, Joint Staff, Geographic Combatant Command, Service headquarters)?
Would you please describe your current position as well as any GHE-related responsibilities or interests related to this position?
How many years of GHE-related experience do you have? Would you briefly describe this experience?
Have you received any GHE-related training and education? If so, who was the provider? In what ways has this training and education helped you in carrying out subsequent GHE responsibilities? In what ways has it been insufficient? Examples would be helpful.

GENERAL QUESTIONS

- From your perspective, what are DoD's (or your CCMD's) top GHE priorities?
- How and to what extent do GHE priorities support global and theater objectives?
- What are the primary types of GHE capabilities that DoD and the CCMDs are seeking to develop over the long term?

- What challenges, if any, do you see in enabling long-term support of GHE-related CCMD objectives?

FUNDING QUESTIONS

- What types of GHE activities are you currently conducting or overseeing?
- Who are your primary governmental partners in planning, resourcing, or executing these activities?
- What are the primary authorities and sources of funding used to support these GHE activities?
- What challenges, if any, are the CCMDs and GHE providers facing in using current authorities and funding sources? What can't they do based on the authority or funding limitations, if anything?
- If some changes are required, what types of funding mechanisms would more effectively support CCMD objectives?
- Do you currently track GHE activities and funding? If so, how? Is this system working well for your office? If not, what changes would you suggest, if any?

CONCLUDING QUESTIONS

- Is there anything else we did not cover that we should consider?
- Are there any other individuals or organizations you feel we should speak to who have good visibility on these issues and could provide valuable insights for our study? Would you kindly provide their contact information?
- Is there any documentation you could share with us that you think would be relevant?

Abbreviations

AFAFRICA	U.S. Air Forces Africa
AFCENT	U.S. Air Forces Central
AFRICOM	U.S. Africa Command
AFSOUTH	U.S. Air Forces Southern
APRI	Asia Pacific Regional Initiative
APRRP	African Peacekeeping Rapid Response Partnership
BPC	building partner capacity
BTRP	Biological Threat Reduction Program
CASEVAC	casualty evacuation
CBA	capabilities-based assessment
CENTCOM	U.S. Central Command
COVID-19	coronavirus disease 2019
DASD	Deputy Assistant Secretary of Defense
DHP	Defense Health Program
DoD	U.S. Department of Defense
DOTmLPF-P	Doctrine, Organization, Training, materiel, Leadership and education, Personnel, Facilities, and Policy
DSCA	Defense Security Cooperation Agency
DTRA	Defense Threat Reduction Agency
EDI	European Deterrence Initiative
EUCOM	U.S. European Command
FMF	Foreign Military Financing
FMS	Foreign Military Sales
GCC	geographic combatant command
GHE	global health engagement
GP	Global Partnerships
GPOI	Global Peace Operations Initiative
HCA	Humanitarian and Civic Assistance
IMET	International Military Education and Training
INDOPACOM	U.S. Indo-Pacific Command
MARFORPAC	U.S. Marine Corps Forces, Pacific
MEDEVAC	medical evacuation
MEDRETE	Medical Readiness Training Exercise
NATO	North Atlantic Treaty Organization
O&M	Operation and Maintenance

OASD	Office of the Assistant Secretary of Defense
OCO	Overseas Contingency Operations
OHDACA	Overseas Humanitarian, Disaster, and Civic Aid
PACAF	U.S. Air Forces Pacific
PACFLT	U.S. Pacific Fleet
PDI	Pacific Deterrence Initiative
PEPFAR	President's Emergency Plan for AIDS Relief
PKO	Peacekeeping Operations
PREACT	Partnership for Regional East Africa Counterterrorism
SOCOM	U.S. Special Operations Command
SOUTHCOM	U.S. Southern Command
SPP	State Partnership Program
TCA	Traditional Combatant Command Activities
TSCTP	Trans-Sahara Counterterrorism Partnership
UAE	United Arab Emirates
USAFE	U.S. Air Forces Europe
USARPAC	U.S. Army Pacific
USUHS	Uniformed Services University of the Health Sciences
WIF	Wales Initiative Fund

References

12th Air Force, "Medical Readiness Training Exercises (MEDRETEs)," webpage, undated. As of March 9, 2022:
https://www.12af.acc.af.mil/About-Us/Fact-Sheets/Display/Article/319237/medical-readiness-training-exercises-medretes/

AFRICOM—*See* U.S. Africa Command.

Beadling, Charles W., "AFRICOM Health Engagement and Security: Beyond Hearts and Minds," Uniformed Services University of the Health Sciences, June 20, 2017. As of April 14, 2022:
http://specialoperationsmedicine.org/Documents/2017%20SOMSA/2017%20Presentations/24May17%201400%20African%20Health%20Engagements%20Charles%20Beadling.pdf

Belkin, Paul, and Hibbah Kaileh, "The European Deterrence Initiative: A Budgetary Overview," Congressional Research Service, IF10946, July 1, 2021.

Bumgardner, Richard, "Medical Ties Bind Forces in Partnership," *Army Magazine*, Vol. 70, No. 8, August 2020.

Cause IQ, "Henry M Jackson Foundation for the Advancement of Military Medicine," webpage, undated. As of July 22, 2022:
https://www.causeiq.com/organizations/henry-m-jackson-foundation-for-the-advancement-of,521317896/

Center for Army Lessons Learned, *Security Cooperation and the State Partnership Program*, October 2018. As of April 19, 2022:
https://usacac.army.mil/sites/default/files/publications/19-01%20State%20Partnership%20Program%20%28Lo%20Res%29.pdf

Center for Global Health Engagement, "2020 Annual Report," 2020. As of March 11, 2022:
https://cghe.usuhs.edu/sites/default/files/media/documents/2020_cghe_annual_report.pdf.pdf

Defense Health Agency, "Department of Defense HIV/AIDS Prevention Program," webpage, undated. As of December 1, 2022:
https://www.health.mil/Military-Health-Topics/Health-Readiness/Public-Health/DHAPP

Defense Security Cooperation Agency, "Foreign Military Sales (FMS)," webpage, undated-a. As of April 13, 2022:
https://www.dsca.mil/foreign-military-sales-fms

Defense Security Cooperation Agency, "Overseas Humanitarian, Disaster, and Civic Aid (OHDACA)," webpage, undated-b. As of August 30, 2021:
https://samm.dsca.mil/chapter/chapter-12

Defense Security Cooperation Agency, "Section 333 Authority to Build Capacity," webpage, undated-c. As of June 13, 2022:
https://www.dsca.mil/section-333-authority-build-capacity

Defense Security Cooperation Agency, "Updates to the Program Codes for the Global Peacekeeping Operations Initiative (GPOI), Peacekeeping Operations (PKO) and Peacekeeping Operations African Peacekeeping Rapid Response Partnership (PKO/APRRP) Programs, DSCA Policy 19-41 [E-Change 444]," memorandum to the Deputy Assistant Secretary of the Army for Defense Exports and Cooperation, Deputy Assistant Secretary of the Navy for International Programs, and Deputy Under Secretary of the Air Force for International Affairs, September 23, 2019a.

Defense Security Cooperation Agency, "Croatia—UH-60M Black Hawk Helicopters," Transmittal No. 19-72, October 30, 2019b. As of April 13, 2022:
https://www.dsca.mil/sites/default/files/mas/croatia_19-72.pdf

Defense Security Cooperation Agency, "Fiscal Year (FY) 2021 Budget Estimates: Operation and Maintenance, Defense-Wide, Overseas Humanitarian, Disaster, and Civic Aid," February 2020. As of August 30, 2021:
https://comptroller.defense.gov/Portals/45/Documents/defbudget/fy2021/budget_justification/pdfs/01_Operation_and_Maintenance/O_M_VOL_1_PART_2/OHDACA_OCO_OP-5.pdf

Defense Security Cooperation University, *Security Cooperation Programs Handbook for Fiscal Year 2020*, 2020.

Defense Security Cooperation University, *Security Cooperation Programs Handbook for Fiscal Year 2021*, 2021.

Defense Security Cooperation University, *Security Cooperation Management*, 42nd ed., 2022. As of December 1, 2022:
https://www.dscu.edu/m/green-book

Department of Defense Directive 2060.02, *DoD Countering Weapons of Mass Destruction (WMD) Policy*, U.S. Department of Defense, January 27, 2017.

Department of Defense Directive 3000.05, *Stabilization*, U.S. Department of Defense, December 13, 2018.

Department of Defense Directive 3000.07, *Irregular Warfare (IW)*, U.S. Department of Defense, Incorporating Change 1, May 12, 2017.

Department of Defense Directive 5100.46, *Foreign Disaster Relief (FDR)*, U.S. Department of Defense, Incorporating Change 1, July 28, 2017.

Department of Defense Directive 6200.04, *Force Health Protection (FHP)*, U.S. Department of Defense, April 23, 2007.

Department of Defense Instruction 2000.30, *Global Health Engagement (GHE) Activities*, U.S. Department of Defense, July 12, 2017.

Department of Defense Instruction 2205.02, *Humanitarian and Civic Assistance (HCA) Activities*, U.S. Department of Defense, Incorporating Change 1, May 22, 2017. As of April 27, 2022:
https://www.esd.whs.mil/Portals/54/Documents/DD/issuances/dodi/220502p.pdf

Department of Defense Instruction 3216.02, *Protection of Human Subjects and Adherence to Ethical Standards in DoD-Conducted and -Supported Research*, U.S. Department of Defense, April 15, 2020.

DoD—*See* U.S. Department of Defense.

EUCOM—*See* U.S. European Command.

Eversden, Andrew, "Pacific Deterrence Initiative Gets $2.1 Billion Boost in Final NDAA," *Breaking Defense*, December 7, 2021. As of March 7, 2022:
https://breakingdefense.com/2021/12/pacific-deterrence-initiative-gets-2-1-billion-boost-in-final-ndaa/

Faller, Craig S., "A Collective Presence in the Western Hemisphere Reduces Threats to the US and Its Allies," *Defense News*, September 5, 2019. As of April 21, 2022:
https://www.defensenews.com/opinion/commentary/2019/09/05/a-collective-presence-in-the-western-hemisphere-reduces-threats-to-the-us-and-its-allies/

Global Health Security Agenda, "About the GHSA," webpage, undated. As of February 9, 2021:
https://ghsagenda.org/about-the-ghsa/

Global Health Security Agenda, *Strengthening Health Security Across the Globe: Progress and Impact of U.S. Government Investments in the Global Health Security Agenda*, October 2021.

Grill, Beth, Michael J. McNerney, Jeremy Boback, Renanah Miles, Cynthia C. Clapp-Wincek, and David E. Thaler, *Follow the Money: Promoting Greater Transparency in Department of Defense Security Cooperation Reporting*, RAND Corporation, RR-2039-OSD, 2017. As of March 29, 2022:
https://www.rand.org/pubs/research_reports/RR2039.html

Jackson, Andrew, "Guam, Hawaii Share COVID Best Practices with the Philippines," National Guard, December 10, 2020. As of April 14, 2022:
https://www.nationalguard.mil/News/State-Partnership-Program/Article/2442114/guam-hawaii-share-covid-best-practices-with-the-philippines/

Joint Publication 1-06, *Financial Management in Joint Operations*, Joint Chiefs of Staff, January 11, 2018. As of April 12, 2022:
https://www.jcs.mil/Portals/36/Documents/Doctrine/pubs/jp1_06pa.pdf?ver=2018-02-08-091410-513

Joint Publication 3-29, *Foreign Humanitarian Assistance*, Joint Chiefs of Staff, May 14, 2019. As of April 27, 2022:
https://www.jcs.mil/Portals/36/Documents/Doctrine/pubs/jp3_29.pdf

Joint Publication 4-02, *Joint Health Services*, Joint Chiefs of Staff, Incorporating Change 1, September 28, 2018. As of December 1, 2022:
https://www.jcs.mil/Portals/36/Documents/Doctrine/pubs/jp4_02ch1.pdf

Jones, Grady, "AFRICOM Africa Malaria Taskforce Key Leader Event–2019 Comes to a Close," U.S. Africa Command, April 15, 2019.

Kaiser Family Foundation, "Breaking Down the U.S. Global Health Budget by Program Area," fact sheet, September 2022.

Kelly, Terrence K., Jefferson P. Marquis, Cathryn Quantic Thurston, Jennifer D. P. Moroney, and Charlotte Lynch, *Security Cooperation Organizations in the Country Team: Options for Success*, RAND Corporation, TR-734-A, 2010. As of December 1, 2022:
https://www.rand.org/pubs/technical_reports/TR734.html

Kline, Mikaley, "Pacific Angel Provides Aid, Builds Partnerships Throughout Indo-Pacific Communities," U.S. Indo-Pacific Command, October 1, 2019. As of March 7, 2022:
https://www.pacom.mil/Media/News/News-Article-View/Article/1976797/pacific-angel-provides-aid-builds-partnerships-throughout-indo-pacific-communit/

Licina, Derek, and Jackson Taylor, "International Trauma Capacity Building Programs: Modernizing Capabilities, Enhancing Lethality, Supporting Alliances, Building Partnerships, and Implementing Reform," *Military Medicine*, Vol. 187, No. 7–8, July–August 2022.

Lykke, Arthur F., Jr., "A Methodology for Developing a Military Strategy," in Arthur F. Lykke, Jr., ed., *Military Strategy: Theory and Application*, U.S. Army War College, 1993.

Manzano, Jesse, "Florida Guard Partners with Guyana to Boost Medical Readiness," National Guard, March 9, 2020. As of April 14, 2022:
https://www.nationalguard.mil/News/State-Partnership-Program/Article/2105381/florida-guard-partners-with-guyana-to-boost-medical-readiness/

Marquis, Jefferson P., Trupti Brahmbhatt, Aaron Clark-Ginsberg, Victoria M. Smith, and David E. Thaler, *Educating and Training the Department of Defense Workforce for Global Health Engagement to Support the Geographic Combatant Commands*, RAND Corporation, RR-A1357-1, 2023. As of June 2023:
https://www.rand.org/pubs/research_reports/RRA1357-1.html

Marshall, Sarah, "Global Health Engagement: The African Peacekeeping Rapid Response Partnership," *The Pulse*, Uniformed Services University blog, March 5, 2018. As of December 1, 2022:
https://usupulse.blogspot.com/2018/03/global-health-engagement-african.html

Mendez, Bryce H. P., "FY2022 Budget Request for the Military Health System," Congressional Research Service, IF11856, June 15, 2021.

Michaud, Josh, Kellie Moss, and Jennifer Kates, *The U.S. Department of Defense and Global Health: Technical Volume*, Kaiser Family Foundation, September 2012. As of October 10, 2021:
https://www.kff.org/global-health-policy/report/the-u-s-department-of-defense-global/

Mniedlo, Rafal, "Allied Spirit Medical Evacuation (MEDEVAC) Training in Poland," U.S. Army Europe and Africa, June 6, 2020. As of March 14, 2022:
https://www.europeafrica.army.mil/Newsroom/Photos/igphoto/2002311944/

Moss, Kellie, and Jennifer Kates, "PEPFAR Reauthorization: Side-by-Side of Legislation over Time," Kaiser Family Foundation, January 29, 2019. As of April 14, 2022:
https://www.kff.org/global-health-policy/issue-brief/pepfar-reauthorization-side-by-side-of-existing-and-proposed-legislation/

Moss, Kellie, and Josh Michaud, *The U.S. Department of Defense and Global Health: Infectious Disease Efforts*, Kaiser Family Foundation, October 2013.

Nash, Gregory, "Multinational Medics, Civilian First Responders 'Save Lives' at Exercise Cope North 2020," U.S. Air Force, March 2, 2020. As of March 7, 2022:
https://www.af.mil/News/Article-Display/Article/2099155/multinational-medics-civilian-first-responders-save-lives-at-exercise-cope-nort/

National Guard, "State Partnership Program," fact sheet, undated. As of December 1, 2022:
https://www.nationalguard.mil/Portals/31/Resources/Fact%20Sheets/State%20Partnership%20Program%20(SPP)%20Fact%20Sheet%2007082022.pdf

NATO—*See* North Atlantic Treaty Organization.

NATO Centre of Excellence for Military Medicine, "Vigorous Warrior," webpage, undated. As of March 7, 2022:
https://www.coemed.org/resources/vw

North Atlantic Treaty Organization, *NATO Logistics Handbook*, 3rd ed., October 1997. As of December 1, 2022:
https://www.nato.int/docu/logi-en/logist97.htm

Office of the Under Secretary of Defense (Comptroller), *European Deterrence Initiative: Department of Defense Budget Fiscal Year (FY) 2020*, March 2019. As of April 21, 2022:
https://comptroller.defense.gov/Portals/45/Documents/defbudget/fy2020/fy2020_EDI_JBook.pdf

Office of the Under Secretary of Defense (Comptroller), *Defense Health Program: Fiscal Year (FY) 2021 Budget Estimates*, February 2020a. As of April 21, 2022:
https://comptroller.defense.gov/Portals/45/Documents/defbudget/fy2021/budget_justification/pdfs/09_Defense_Health_Program/Defense_Health_Program_fy2021_Budget_Estimates.pdf

Office of the Under Secretary of Defense (Comptroller), *European Deterrence Initiative: Department of Defense Budget Fiscal Year (FY) 2021*, February 2020b. As of April 12, 2022:
https://comptroller.defense.gov/Portals/45/Documents/defbudget/FY2021/FY2021_EDI_JBook.pdf

Office of the Under Secretary of Defense (Comptroller), "Fiscal Year (FY) 2021 Budget Estimates: Operation and Maintenance, Defense-Wide, Cooperative Threat Reduction Program," February 2020c. As of April 11, 2022:
https://comptroller.defense.gov/Portals/45/Documents/defbudget/fy2021/budget_justification/pdfs/01_Operation_and_Maintenance/O_M_VOL_1_PART_2/CTR_OP-5.pdf

Office of the Under Secretary of Defense (Comptroller), "Fiscal Year (FY) 2021 Budget Estimates: Operation and Maintenance, Defense-Wide, The Joint Staff," February 2020d. As of April 11, 2022:
https://comptroller.defense.gov/Portals/45/Documents/defbudget/fy2021/budget_justification/pdfs/01_Operation_and_Maintenance/O_M_VOL_1_PART_1/TJS_OP-5.pdf

Office of the Under Secretary of Defense (Comptroller), "Fiscal Year 2022 President's Budget: Defense Security Cooperation Agency," May 2021. As of April 12, 2022:
https://comptroller.defense.gov/Portals/45/Documents/defbudget/fy2022/budget_justification/pdfs/01_Operation_and_Maintenance/O_M_VOL_1_PART_1/DSCA_OP-5.pdf

Office of the Under Secretary of Defense (Comptroller), *European Deterrence Initiative: Department of Defense Budget Fiscal Year (FY) 2023*, April 2022. As of July 8, 2022:
https://comptroller.defense.gov/Portals/45/Documents/defbudget/FY2023/FY2023_EDI_JBook.pdf

Office of the Under Secretary of Defense (Comptroller) and Chief Financial Officer, *Defense Budget Overview: United States Department of Defense Fiscal Year 2023 Budget Request*, April 2022. As of July 8, 2022:
https://comptroller.defense.gov/Portals/45/Documents/defbudget/FY2023/FY2023_Budget_Request_Overview_Book.pdf

Perez, Casey, Diana Aguirre, Brian Neese, Joshua Vess, and Edwin K. Burkett, "Evaluating Team Characteristics for Health Engagements in Three Countries in Central America: 2012–2017," *Military Medicine*, July 6, 2021.

Public Law 111-118, Department of Defense Appropriations Act, 2010; Section 8094, December 19, 2009.

Public Law 115-31, Consolidated Appropriations Act, 2017, May 5, 2017.

Public Law 117-103, Consolidated Appropriations Act, 2022; Section 8042, Humanitarian Assistance, March 15, 2022.

Schwier-Morales, Armando A., "USAFE Offers Knowledge to Polish Flying Doctors," Air Force Medical Service, December 7, 2015. As of March 14, 2022:
https://www.airforcemedicine.af.mil/News/Article/633870/usafe-offers-knowledge-to-polish-flying-doctors/

Selva, Paul, Vice Chairman of the Joint Chiefs of Staff, "DOTmLPF-P Change Recommendation for Global Health Engagement," memorandum, JROCM 008-19, February 25, 2019, Not available to the general public.

Serafino, Nina M., *The Global Peace Operations Initiative: Background and Issues for Congress*, Congressional Research Service, June 11, 2009.

SOUTHCOM—*See* U.S. Southern Command.

Thaler, David E., Michael J. McNerney, Beth Grill, Jefferson P. Marquis, and Amanda Kadlec, *From Patchwork to Framework: A Review of Title 10 Authorities for Security Cooperation*, RAND Corporation, RR-1438-OSD, 2016. As of March 29, 2022:
https://www.rand.org/pubs/research_reports/RR1438.html

Thomas, Brent, *Preparing for the Future of Combat Casualty Care: Opportunities to Refine the Military Health System's Alignment with the National Defense Strategy*, RAND Corporation, RR-A713-1, 2021. As of March 29, 2022:
https://www.rand.org/pubs/research_reports/RRA713-1.html

Torres Chardon, Juan, "Crews Provide Aeromedical Evacuation Capabilities in Cope North Exercise," U.S. Department of Defense, February 28, 2018. As of March 9, 2022:
https://www.defense.gov/News/News-Stories/Article/Article/1454277/crews-provide-aeromedical-evacuation-capabilities-in-cope-north-exercise/

Uniformed Services University, "Department of Defense Global Health Engagement," briefing, undated.

Uniformed Services University Center for Global Health Engagement, "Programs and Operational Support," webpage, undated. As of April 20, 2022:
https://cghe.usuhs.edu/programs

U.S. Africa Command, "AFRICOM'S Health Engagements," briefing, September 4, 2019, Not available to the general public.

U.S. Africa Command, "AFRICOM's Partnership Endures During COVID-19," April 14, 2020. As of April 20, 2022:
https://www.africom.mil/pressrelease/32693/africoms-partnership-endures-during-covid-19

U.S. Army Pacific, "FY21 Health Security Cooperation/Global Health Engagement OAIs," undated, Not available to the general public.

U.S. Army Pacific Surgeon's Office, "Health Theater Security Cooperation/Global Health Engagement Deep Dive," briefing, September 2020.

USARPAC—See U.S. Army Pacific.

U.S. Code, Title 10, Section 166a, Combatant Commands: Funding Through the Chairman of Joint Chiefs of Staff.

U.S. Code, Title 10, Section 333, Foreign Security Forces: Authority to Build Capacity.

U.S. Code, Title 10, Section 1100, Defense Health Program Account.

U.S. Code, Title 10, Section 2561, Humanitarian Assistance.

U.S. Code, Title 50, Section 3711, Authority to Carry Out Department of Defense Cooperative Threat Reduction Program.

U.S. Department of Defense, *The State Partnership Program: FY2015 Annual Report to Congress*, December 2016.

U.S. Department of Defense, *Global Health Engagement (GHE) Capabilities-Based Assessment (CBA) Study*, July 23, 2018, Not available to the general public.

U.S. Department of Defense, *Non-Program of Record U.S. Industry Handbook*, July 2020.

U.S. Department of Defense, "2022 Learning and Evaluation Agenda for Partnerships Framework," August 25, 2022.

U.S. Department of Defense, Military Health System, "Combat Support," webpage, undated-a. As of June 13, 2022:
https://www.health.mil/Military-Health-Topics/Combat-Support

U.S. Department of Defense, Military Health System, "Global Health Engagement," webpage, undated-b. As of April 20, 2022:
https://www.health.mil/Military-Health-Topics/Health-Readiness/Global-Health-Engagement

U.S. Department of Defense Office of Inspector General, *Audit of U.S. Africa Command's Execution of Coronavirus Aid, Relief, and Economic Security Act Funding*, March 31, 2022. As of April 20, 2022:
https://media.defense.gov/2022/Apr/04/2002968941/-1/-1/1/DODIG-2022-080.PDF

U.S. Department of State, "Key Topics—Office of Global Programs and Initiatives," webpage, undated-a. As of April 20, 2022:
https://www.state.gov/key-topics-office-of-global-programs-and-initiatives/

U.S. Department of State, "The United States President's Emergency Plan for AIDS Relief," webpage, undated-b. As of April 13, 2022:
https://www.state.gov/pepfar/

U.S. Department of State, "U.S. Peacekeeping Capacity Building Assistance," fact sheet, May 27, 2022. As of July 22, 2022:
https://www.state.gov/u-s-peacekeeping-capacity-building-assistance/

U.S. Department of State Bureau of Counterterrorism, "Programs and Initiatives," webpage, undated. As of April 13, 2022:
https://www.state.gov/bureau-of-counterterrorism-programs-and-initiatives/

U.S. Embassy in Rwanda, "Handover Ceremony of the AMEP Medical Modeling and Simulation Project," February 7, 2016. As of April 14, 2022:
https://rw.usembassy.gov/ambassador-amep/

U.S. European Command, "FY 2020 European Deterrence Initiative (EDI) Fact Sheet," undated. As of April 12, 2022:
https://www.eucom.mil/document/39921/fy-2020-european-deterrence-initiative-fact-s

U.S. European Command, *EUCOM Combatant Command Campaign Plan 2018: Health Security Cooperation*, May 15, 2018, Appendix 3 to Annex Q, Not available to the general public.

U.S. European Command, *EUCOM Combatant Command Campaign Plan 2020: Global Health Engagement*, 2021, Appendix 10 to Annex Q, Not available to the general public.

U.S. European Command Global Health Engagement Working Group, briefing, August 12, 2020, Not available to the general public.

U.S. Government Accountability Office, *Influenza Pandemic: DOD Combatant Commands'
Preparedness Efforts Could Benefit from More Clearly Defined Roles, Resources, and Risk
Mitigation*, GAO-07-696, June 2007. As of December 1, 2022:
https://www.gao.gov/products/gao-07-696

U.S. Government Accountability Office, *Combating Terrorism: State Department Can Improve
Management of East Africa Program*, GAO-14-502, June 2014a. As of April 13, 2022:
https://www.gao.gov/products/gao-14-502

U.S. Government Accountability Office, *Combating Terrorism: U.S. Efforts in Northwest Africa
Would Be Strengthened by Enhanced Program Management*, GAO-14-518, June 2014b. As
of April 14, 2022:
https://www.gao.gov/products/gao-14-518

U.S. Government Accountability Office, *President's Emergency Plan for Aids Relief: State
Should Improve Data Quality and Assess Long-Term Resource Needs*, GAO-21-374, May
2021. As of December 1, 2022:
https://www.gao.gov/products/gao-21-374

U.S. House of Representatives, Global Health Security Act of 2021, Bill 391, July 12, 2021. As
of March 7, 2022:
https://www.congress.gov/bill/117th-congress/house-bill/391/text

U.S. Senate, *Department of Defense Authorization for Appropriations for Fiscal Year 2018 and
the Future Years Defense Program*, hearing before the Senate Committee on Armed
Services, U.S. Government Publishing Office, 2020. As of April 13, 2022:
https://www.govinfo.gov/content/pkg/CHRG-115shrg39567/pdf/CHRG-115shrg39567.pdf

U.S. Southern Command, "A Partnership Approach to Global Health Engagements," briefing,
undated, Not available to the general public.

U.S. Southern Command, "U.S. Military Wraps Up Disaster Relief Exercise in Belize," January
18, 2022. As of March 13, 2022:
https://www.southcom.mil/MEDIA/NEWS-ARTICLES/Article/2902562/us-military-wraps-
up-disaster-relief-exercise-in-belize/

Vedula, Padmaja, Trupti Brahmbhatt, Jonathan Tran, and Chandler Sachs, *Assessing Technology
Platforms for Global Health Engagement to Support Integration of Efforts Across
Geographic Combatant Commands*, RAND Corporation, RR-A1357-3, 2023. As of June
2023:
https://www.rand.org/pubs/research_reports/RRA1357-3.html

Vergun, David, "DOD Supports Partner Nations with COVID-19 Mitigation Assistance," U.S. Department of Defense, June 1, 2020. As of March 14, 2022: https://www.defense.gov/News/News-Stories/Article/Article/2203398/dod-supports-partner-nations-with-covid-19-mitigation-assistance/source/dod-supports-partner-nations-with-covid-19-mitigation-assistance/

Walker, Dustin, "Show Me the Money: Boost the Pacific Deterrence Initiative," *War on the Rocks*, June 29, 2022.

Warner, Lesley Anne, *The Trans Sahara Counter Terrorism Partnership: Building Partner Capacity to Counter Terrorism and Violent Extremism*, CNA, March 2014. As of April 13, 2022: https://www.cna.org/cna_files/pdf/crm-2014-u-007203-final.pdf

The White House, *Indo-Pacific Strategy of the United States*, February 2022.